VITAMIN C . . . WHO NEEDS IT?

VITAMIN C . . . WHO NEEDS IT?

E. Cheraskin, M.D., D.M.D.

Arlington Press & Company • 1993

For information contact June Cunniff at
Arlington Press
2225-A Arlington Avenue
Birmingham, Alabama 35205
205.933.9524 (phone)
205.933.9420 (fax)

ISBN 0–944353–04–5
Printed and bound in the United States of
America.
LSF 1 2 3 4 5 6 7 8 9 10

TABLE OF CONTENTS

IN THE BEGINNING . . .

Vitamin C . . . who needs it!?

Ask different doctors if you should take vitamin C and you'll probably get the same answers one of my patient received 35 years ago. His internist angrily responded, "Absolutely not, it will give you kidney stones." His urologist, in a cavalier style answered, "It doesn't matter, if you don't need it you'll excrete it." And his otorhinolaryngologist insisted, "Definitely, yes, it will help you with your allergies and colds."

He then came to me for a fourth opinion . . . and I still get the same calls, even today.

What's interesting is that with proper studies it should be possible to eliminate the confusion over vitamin C's role in maintaining health. Like oxygen, vitamin C is essential. No argument. Every cell and therefore all tissues, organs, and sites need vitamin C. It follows that if and when this nutrient is properly viewed, it will become clear that all medical conditions and diseases are, to a varying degree, ascorbate dependent. It might be that C will sound like snake oil, a cure for everything! However, as you will learn within these pages, man does not live by C alone.

As hard as it is to imagine, the human organism is actually a bag of electrical charges. Vitamin C is an electron donor. It helps make the cells behave in an orderly fashion.

Much has already been written about the ascorbates. There have been several conferences by the New York Academy of Sciences; two world congresses have appeared under the aegis of Alacer Corporation of California. Our group has published two books. *The Vitamin C Connection* (in hardback by Harper and Row in 1983 and in paperback by Bantam Books in 1984) was intended to show the extraordinary versatility of the ascorbates in lay education language. In 1988, we released *The Vitamin C Controversy: Questions and Answers* (BioCommunications Press) designed to answer the 50 most commonly asked questions regarding our then 82 publications on the subject of vitamin C metabolism.

All of this has required extraordinary support and talent. Never is a book a one-person job. I have been fortunate in working with Sara Gay, my secretary/assistant/partner, without whom this manuscript would never have been possible. I acknowledge associates through these many years who have already been dutifully noted in their respective publications. I wish to take this opportunity to thank Abram Hoffer, M.D., Ph.D., and Steven Carter, of the Canadian Schizophrenia Foundation, for prepublishing the manuscript in serial form in their newsletter, *Health and*

Nutrition Update. This provided us with a superb opportunity to pretest the manuscript. We also here acknowledge the Cunniff Public Relations and Arlington Press for their publisher/printer/media creative and constructive contributions.

Time for a prediction . . . if and when vitamin C is explored with the same enthusiasm, time, and money presently devoted to space research the benefits so derived will underscore the wonders of the ascorbates.

Finally, it is our hope that the reading of this manuscript will reduce or eliminate the need for the second, third and fourth opinions!

1

VITAMIN C ...
WHO NEEDS IT?

Vitamin C ... who needs it?

The quick and honest answer depends on whom you ask.

There are experts who will tell you that vitamin C isn't a critical medical issue. Other authorities will argue that it's a matter of life and death; while yet another group will assume an in-between stance, one of the shades-of-grey. There will be an almost infinite number of so-called expert opinions, with each varied opinion stemming from a different definition derived from a differing perspective.

Picture the following scene:

A doctor's office. The physician has just complet-ed an oration about the merits of the well-known, well-balanced diet. The patient rises, walks to the door, opens it, and then turns to the doctor.

Patient: By the way, Doctor, do you ever encounter any vitamin C problems?

Doctor: No, not really.

Patient: Have you ever thought it necessary to measure vitamin C?

Doctor: No, why?

Patient: Isn't that a good way not to see any problems?

The doctor turns to the audience, baffled, as the curtain falls.

The point is that no modern practitioner would confirm a diagnosis of diabetes **mellitus*** without measuring blood sugar. But, this very same doctor is assured of optimal vitamin C state without even measuring **ascorbic acid** (**AA**). Part of the problem regarding *Vitamin C . . . who needs it?* may rest with different definitions stemming from different (or the lack of) measurement.

Within these pages, I will attempt to answer the question *Vitamin C . . . who needs it?* by examining it from diverse perspectives. What is the answer when viewed from an evolutionary standpoint? What can we learn from history? Do the public health officials have their own concept? Is it the same, or how does it vary, from that of the dietitians? Can one better answer the question from a **biochemical** and/or **physiologic** standpoint? Where does this nutrient fit in the **ecologic** equation for health and sickness?

* *Items included in the glossary are in boldface when they first appear in the text.*

We will examine approximately fifty studies. The common denominator is that all of these experiments will deal with human beings under carefully-supervised conditions. This should not be interpreted to mean that the **double-blind** experience is necessarily the only or the final answer.[1] (By the way, double-blind is a manner of conducting an experiment so as to assure statistically reliable results, with neither experimenter nor subjects knowing what is used.) Additionally, while the studies are not general knowledge, they all have appeared in respectable, scientific, English-language journals. Hence, they are readily available and can be confirmed. All of them are simple, clear, and dramatic so that the results are incontestable.

Here's an example of the type of stories that you will encounter throughout this book.

Every Mom's Nightmare

Not uncommonly, Mother, sooner or later, is panicked by the idea that her Dennis is "too small for his age." Obviously, this makes for a rush to the pediatrician. His comment, more often than not, is "not to worry . . . he'll outgrow it." The simple fact of the matter is that the doctor really doesn't know. He is simply playing the odds.

It is, of course, possible that the problem isn't serious and that Dennis will indeed outgrow it. However, there may be more to the story.

And here it is.

Judy Z. Miller and her associates in the Department of Medical Genetics at Indiana University School of Medicine and colleagues at Eli Lilly and

Company administered vitamin C to one of each of 44 allegedly healthy school-aged **monozygotic** (a fancy word for identical) twins for five months.[2] The other twin was given an indistinguishable (blank) supplement. The purpose of this program was simply to examine in a general way the potential therapeutic effects of the **ascorbates**. One aspect, albeit serendipitous, is germane here. Nobody expected the effect ascorbic acid had on growth of these young male twins. In the seven pairs of the youngest group (6 to 11 years of age), in all but one instance, the treated twin grew from 0.64 to 2.54 centimeters (cm) more than did the placebo-administered subject. Simply put, this means that in less than one-half year, one twin grew as much as one inch taller. And all of this was made possible with about 250 milligrams (mg) of vitamin C twice a day!

We should have known it. The celebrated Professor Sherry Lewin[3] (we'll be hearing more about him later) told us way back in 1976 that **pharmacologic** doses of vitamin C might influence growth. He also indicated that this could be done by either altering the equilibrium between ascorbic acid levels in blood and bone or by stimulating **collagen synthesis**. These and other mechanisms will be explored further in subsequent chapters.

We should have anticipated the Miller experiment. In 1969, our group studied the vitamin C state in apparently healthy youngsters being readied for orthodontic treatment.[4-7] Using diagnostic tests (to be enlarged upon later in Chapter Four), we noted that as many as three out of four of these children could be viewed as being **hypoascorbemic**. We then studied the relationship between their actual or chronologic age versus their biologic or bone age and dental eruption schedule. It became obvious that the children in the most optimal vitamin C state paralleled the most "on time" maturation.

Infertility . . . Who is to Blame?

As recently as 1988, a publication by the Office of Technology Assessment[8] provided the estimate that 8.5% of married couples with wives between the ages of 15 and 44 are infertile. In plain language, this covers approximately 2.4 million families in this country. However, others[9] say the number has climbed from 15 to 18 to 20% in the past decade.

Whatever the figures, it's a sad commentary that, in what should be one of the healthiest and happiest periods of their lives, one in twelve couples cannot have a baby!

As often as not, the woman is blamed. Increasingly, however, the evidence is accumulating that infertility may well be the result of some type of male dysfunction.

And what do we now know?

Fact One: In 1941, researchers recognized that the concentration of vitamin C in the testicle was around 20 times higher than in the blood. This raised the question as to whether this tremendous amount might not be of some functional significance.

Fact Two: Six years later, research investigators noted that a majority of infertile males exhibited a low testicular vitamin C level.

Fact Three: Approximately seven years after

that, the experts discovered that the stickiness of sperm was part of the cause of infertility.

Fact Four: Within the next four years, we learned that making sperm less sticky reduced infertility and that vitamin C aided this process.

Fact Five: We now know that ascorbate can increase sperm volume, count, and motility. It also reduces the number of abnormal sperm and their stickiness. Finally, improved sperm quality follows.

So here is the sequence of events. Harris and his associates[10] provided one gram of ascorbic acid per day (this is roughly 12 glasses of orange juice) for 60 days to 20 clearly-diagnosed infertile, but otherwise healthy, men. A separate control (placebo-supplemented) group consisted of 20 men. At the end of these two months, none of the control group's wives reported pregnancies. However, in all of the vitamin C supplemented group, there was conception!

More than Just Fertility . . . Healthy Babies?

Fine . . . we now know how to insure greater fertility. But the ultimate goal is to guarantee a healthy baby. This is becoming more worrisome because of the increasing evidence of a greater incidence and prevalence of congenital defects.

Can AA invite a healthier offspring?

There was a slight clue earlier. Fact Five mentioned that the ascorbates were in some way related to the quality of the sperm.

A group from the University of California at

Berkeley report their findings in the 15 December 1991 issue of the *Proceedings of the National Academy of Sciences.*[11] These researchers have linked low levels of vitamin C to increased genetic (deoxyribonucleic acid or DNA) damage in sperm. In plain English, the DNA aberrations in sperm presumably translate into a greater risk of genetic distortions in the fertilized embryo. There results an increased chance of birth defects. As a matter of fact, we have here a breakthrough. This is the first study to show a connection between low levels of vitamin C and DNA damage. We will enlarge upon this and many other ascorbate functions in a later discussion (Chapter Five).

But now back to more particulars. Fraza and his colleagues carried out several experiments. In a fertility clinic in Buenos Aires, semen samples were obtained from 24 men. These researchers analyzed vitamin C levels in the seminal fluid and the number of chemical modifications in sperm DNA. They found that in men with vitamin C levels below a certain point (corresponding to about 50 or 60 mgs of dietary ascorbic acid per day) DNA damage increased significantly.

The upper ranges of vitamin C intake looked at in this study are about what a person would get by following the dietary recommendations of the National Cancer Institute and the U.S. Department of Agriculture, namely two servings of fruit and three servings of vegetables per day.

How common is this level of intake? According to *Time* (6 April 1992):[12]

. . . a mere 9% of adults manage to consume five servings of fruits and vegetables each day according to the National Center for Health Statistics.

Making Healthy Kids Healthier . . .

For most of us, health/sickness is a black and white, either/or concept. By this definition, making healthy kids healthier is a contradiction in terms. Most of us (including our health experts), by act if not by word, assume that the majority of children are healthy. Unless the youngster has brittle diabetes, the swollen joints of classical rheumatic fever, or a glaring congenital defect, we take it for granted that there is health.

But, for the purists, health/sickness represents a spectrum ranging from health (white) to disease and death (black) with an infinite number of intermediate gradations. There is, in fact, average health (outlined just above) versus optimal, ideal, and possibly perfect health. It now becomes conceivable for healthy kids to be made healthier.

Five investigators from Zagreb, in the former Republic of Yugoslavia,[13] looked beyond this traditional concept. They sought the acme (the ultimate in health) through a continuing series of vitamin studies extending over a number of years. One phase emphasized the effect of ascorbic acid supplementation on physical working capacity in adolescent boys. After daily administration for two months of 70 mg ascorbic acid, the **mean** plasma vitamin C in the 49 subjects in the experimental group rose four and one-half fold. There was a bonus of improved oxygen utilization. No convincing changes in biochemical state or in oxygen consumption could be shown in the 42 placebo-supplemented children. Hence, according to Suboticanec-Buzina and his Yugoslavian colleagues from the Department of Nutrition at the Institute of Public

Health, it's clear that overall performance can be heightened even in seemingly healthy kids.

There is much more to the story. Some of it will appear in subsequent chapters. For our purposes, one vitamin C expert (Doctor C.A.B. Clemetson, author of a monumental three-volume review of the subject) best describes the picture:[14]

> Clearly, about half the boys in the supplemented group showed a very marked increase in working capacity, such as would likely make the difference between losing and winning their next soccer game. Moreover, their improved ascorbate status could lift their spirits and would most probably improve their resistance to infection.

Is it Always Tired (Iron-Poor) Blood?

In our present culture, anemia conjures up an image of a woman with iron-poor blood. If this turns out not to be the case, then she's pigeonholed with a psychiatric/psychologic label.

Need this be so?

The unique role of AA in **intermediary metabolism** is well-established. It will be dealt with in greater detail later (Chapter Five). We know vitamin C plays a role in the formation and maintenance of certain essential blood components (**haemoglobin, hematocrit, red blood cells**).

To test these relationships, two Nigerian researchers carried out a simple and well-supervised study of 32 apparently healthy female nursing students, aged 20 to 34 years.[15] The subjects were randomly divided into three categories. Group A received 100 mg of ascorbic acid, the second subset (B) was given 50 mg per diem. Group C served as the control. They first examined the nurses' hematologic picture initially, then after eight weeks of supplementation, and finally ten weeks after withdrawal. Following both levels of vitamin C administration, there was a significant and favorable response in haemoglobin, hematocrit and **red blood cell count**. This incidentally paralleled a rise in the plasma and white cell ascorbate level. Ten weeks after withdrawal of the supplements, values for all parameters decreased significantly to initial baselines.

The point of the story is obvious. In healthy young women, favorable and desirable changes in the blood picture are possible with relatively small amounts of ascorbate supplementation during a surprisingly short period of time.

How Did We Get into the Act?

Our group at the University of Alabama at Birmingham began a lovefest with vitamin C back in the 1950s. We are often asked how it all came to pass. The first and usual answer is that we knew then in the 50s that you would be asking this question of us in the 90s . . . so we thought it best to get ready! The fact of the matter is that we have no idea how we were mesmerized enough with ascorbic acid to begin this 40+ year journey.

True, we have had a long and abiding interest in measurement. You may recall the earlier scene in the physician's office. It seemed to us that one of the first issues with regard to vitamin C was to measure the us to study AA in the skin. A five-part series resulted entitled *The Intradermal Ascorbic Acid Test.*[16-20] Since then we have published several score of papers on the subject. In 1983, we released *The Vitamin C Connection.*[21] This book was designed for lay-educational purposes. More recently, we compiled a technical report, *The Vitamin C Controversy: Questions and Answers,*[22] intended to capture our responses to the 50 most commonly asked questions of us about the then 82 papers we had released on the subject of vitamin C.

And Now . . . A Vindication

In any case, we did get involved and happily so because the evidence now supports a continuing and burgeoning public as well as professional interest. In this regard, it is now a matter of record that in 1980, 35% of the adult population consumed supplementary vitamin C. Ascorbate was taken by more than 90% of all supplement users. What is particularly noteworthy is the median intake was three times greater than the Recommended Dietary Allowances (RDAs), a subject to be dealt with in Chapter Three.

From a commercial standpoint, the bottom line has now been proclaimed by the Council for Responsible Nutrition in Washington, D.C. We learned from them that, for the past four years, the total sales for over-the-counter (nonprescription) multivitamin/mineral preparations was approximately two billion dollars. Of that amount, vitamin C swallows up 12.3% . . . one in eight dollars!

The hottest news comes from the 1991 *Prevention Magazine* survey.[23] From their analysis of 5,000 readers (obviously health enthusiasts), vitamin C is reported as the number one preparation for the prevention of colds and other infections (78%). Number four (or 76%) is once again vitamin C to reduce the symptoms and/or durations of the common cold. (We had best bear this in mind when we discuss infections in Chapter Six.) The same survey emphasizes the use of the ascorbates for gingival bleeding (77%). (This will pop up again in Chapter Nine.) Finally, 72% of the respondents also recognized the value of this nutrient in the solution of circulatory problems (Chapter Seven).

Summary and Conclusions

We began this discussion by posing the question *Vitamin C . . . who needs it?* We promised answers, not necessarily new, but not well known. And we did just that in this chapter with four simple scientifically-sound studies. For practical purposes and as judged in traditional circles, none of these subjects would have been regarded as ill. Yet under these clearly-controlled conditions, there were striking benefits. In the one case, children seemed to grow taller. In the second instance, infertile but otherwise healthy men resolved their problem. Thirdly, youngsters in an elementary school program clearly showed improvement in work capacity. Finally, asymptomatic nurses netted blood benefits usually associated with the tired blood syndrome.

So, *Vitamin C . . . who needs it?* From these data it appears that subjects ordinarily regarded as healthy can profit by additional vitamin C administration.

2

A LOOK BACK IN TIME

The Anglo-Saxon scurvy (Latin *scorbutis*) is a clinical disorder characterized by extreme weakness, spongy gums, a tendency to develop hemorrhages under the skin and elsewhere due to a deficiency of vitamin C.

This chapter will look into where, why, and how this story began.

Evolutionary Ruminations

The saga begins about fifty (give or take five or ten) million years ago. Obviously, I was not there. Hence, for me, this is all hearsay. However, I have friends who make it sound as if they were there. So, if you can believe my friends who have devoted considerable time studying the subject, then you must accept this tale.

Apparently, humans (or at least our then predecessors) roamed the tropical jungles, interested only in survival which included the constant ingestion of the vitamin C-rich vegetation.

Actually, these early people (like all other animals at that time) were endowed with the machinery to make ascorbic acid. Enzymes in their bodies worked to change glucose into **l-ascorbic acid** through a series of intermediate steps. So humans were lucky; they had choices. They could make vitamin C from sugar. (Even today, the ascorbates are commercially manufactured from glucose.) On the other hand, the alternative was to simply munch on high C foods.

For reasons still unclear, an accident occurred resulting in the genetic elimination of the critical enzyme, l-gulonolactone oxidase, necessary for the last step in the transfer of sugar to ascorbic acid. This created no serious problems. People could resort to the alternative . . . namely to continue eating fruits and vegetables with high ascorbate content.

And so, the human creatures lived happily until (for whatever reasons) they moved to the city. Now they were in trouble. They had lost their vitamin C machinery. Hence, they now had to eat these special foods to live.

In short, we humans are dependent upon vitamin C . . . just as hooked as we are on oxygen. If we were to cut off the air in the room, in a matter of minutes we would die. Before we passed away, during that short period, there would be a few unusual symptoms and signs such as a cherry red complexion, giggling, and with impending unconsciousness, nonsense jabbering.

Similarly, if we were to abruptly discontinue vitamin C intake, we would just as surely die. However,

the demise would occur over months (rather than minutes as with oxygen). Hence, there would be the opportunity to have a considerable number of clinical aberrations such as we've just learned . . . weakness,
spongy gums, and generalized bleeding.

Have we unraveled the evolutionary puzzle? Only
partly. Other investigators have continued to add
pieces. One such researcher is Matthias Rath, M.D. of
the Linus Pauling Institute for Science and Medicine.[1]
He makes the point that a better understanding of the
whole story is possible when one integrates the genetic
factor with metabolic considerations, diet and the environment. This will become more evident in a later discussion (Chapter Seven).

So, *Vitamin C . . . who needs it?* Just as with oxygen, everybody. There ought not to be any question
about that. The argument really centers on how much,
when, and how.

The Explorers' Sickness

Skipping now from evolution to history, at the end
of the Middle Ages, sailors began to make ever more
daring voyages out from western Europe. This could be
explained, in part, by technical developments in the
design of the ships that allowed sailing at a greater
angle from the direction of the wind, and in methods of
navigation with a more reliable compass. There were
also strong commercial inducements to find a more
profitable sea route in lieu of the overland trade of silk
and spices between Europe and the Far East.

We know that Portuguese sailors began to explore
Africa in the 1400s finally rounding the Cape in 1487.
It soon became obvious, though, that on such long voy-

ages sailors became quite ill. Their hands and feet swelled and their gums grew over their teeth, which made eating difficult if not impossible. Quite by accident, a group of sailors encountered Moors who were carrying oranges which seemed to provide a magical cure. (This is another in a series of exciting serendipitous stories which will crop up in later chapters.)

For our purposes, we can skip the subsequent experiences with the French, English and the Dutch. There is ample documentation that their Navies suffered the same fate. All of this is glaringly described in almost all historical accounts of scurvy including the reporting of Kenneth J. Carpenter, a professor of nutrition at the University of California in Berkeley.[2]

The James Lind Experiment

One naval surgeon who became particularly interested in the problem of scurvy at sea was James Lind, now the most celebrated name in the history of this subject. It was during one such outbreak of scurvy that Lind carried out his famous experiment—probably the first controlled trial in clinical nutrition, or even in any branch of clinical science.

He studied a group of sailors all with scurvy under what today would be viewed as an acceptable double-blind study. Without delving into all the particulars, it became evident that this terrible syndrome responded almost magically to the consumption of oranges and lemons.

In 1748, Lind left the Navy and returned to Edinburgh. In 1750, he set out to write a short paper on scurvy for the Society of Naval Surgeons, but it expanded into a 400-page book known now as the celebrated *A Treatise of the Scurvy.*

While the arguments continued to rage at that time (and regrettably still do), British sailors became so convinced that they began to praise in song the virtues of vitamin C:

We were all hearty seamen,
no colds did we fear
And we have from all sickness entirely kept clear
Thanks be to the Captain,
he has proved so good
Amongst all the islands to give us fresh food.

The Dark Ages

As we have just learned, the vitamin C connection was established with the recognition that an absence of what later became known as vitamin C led to a fatal disease identified as scurvy. When the connection was finally and firmly established, the scientific community rested with the happy thought that here was a specific substance associated with a specific syndrome.

From this time on until the middle of the 1900s, not much occurred clinically. True, there were some isolated brilliant discoveries like the identification of vitamin C by Albert Szent-Gyorgyi.[3] However, from a practical clinical standpoint, the two centuries from 1750 to about 1950 could be viewed as the Dark Ages.

The Twentieth Century
Wake-up Calls

While the initial connection, as we have seen, was identified years ago, the notion of a bigger and better connection is relatively new. Since the 1950s many excellent and highly imaginative contributions have been made.

Irwin Stone deserves much credit for having marshalled the arguments that indicate that most human beings have been receiving amounts of ascorbic acid lower than those required to put them in the best of health. It is his contention and supported by much evidence, (mentioned earlier in this chapter) that most people in this world have a disease involving a deficient intake of ascorbic acid, a disorder that he's named **hypoascorbemia**. It's possible that most people in the world receive only one or two percent of the amounts of vitamin C that would keep them in the best of health. The resulting suboptimal C state may be responsible for many of the illnesses that plague mankind. Doctor Stone's work summarizes the evidence in a book entitled *The Healing Factor.*[4]

One of the most exciting (and by the way another serendipitous) piece of this story comes to us from Professor Linus Pauling:

> In April 1966, I received a letter from Dr. Irwin Stone, a biochemist whom I had met at the Carl Neuberg Medal Award dinner in New York the previous month. He mentioned in his letter that I had expressed a desire to live for the next 15 or 20 years . . . . He accordingly was sending me a description of his high-level ascorbic acid regimen . . . . My wife and I began the regimen recommended by Dr. Stone. We noticed an increased feeling of well-being, and especially a striking decrease in the number of colds that we caught, and in their severity.

As the record now shows, Doctor Pauling became fascinated with the potential of vitamin C in this seemingly **nonscorbutic** area. This led to his books on the common cold[5] and influenza[6] which created both a professional and public furor.

The story now shifts to Scotland. Doctor Ewan Cameron, a surgeon with a long interest in the treatment of cancer patients, became convinced that the most important factor determining the progress and outcome of any cancer illness is the natural resistance of the patient to his or her disease. In his 1966 book, *Hyaluronidase and Cancer*,[7] he pointed out that the resistance of the normal tissues surrounding a malignant tumor to infiltration by the malignancy would be increased if the strength of the intercellular cement (also called ground substance) that binds the cells of the normal tissues together could be increased.

It is in fact known that some, and probably all, malignant **neoplasms** liberate an enzyme, hyaluronidase, that causes the cement to be cut into smaller molecules. This weakens the basic ground substance. Moreover, some, and perhaps all, malignant tumors also liberate another enzyme, collagenase, that causes the **collagen fibrils** to be split into small molecules, further weakening the normal tissues making the cancer spread easier.

Ewan Cameron . . . collagen . . . vitamin C . . . enter Linus Pauling . . . all of this resulted in *Cancer and Vitamin C*.[8]

Prior to Pauling/Cameron/Stone, during and since those days, there have been many investigators who have published extensively on the relationship of vitamin C to seemingly nonscorbutic syndromes. Many of these studies will constitute the bulk of the rest of this monograph.

We here at the University of Alabama Medical

Center, as pointed out earlier, became interested in the 1950s, concentrating our efforts in a number of areas. We produced a series of reports on the quantification of vitamin C utilizing generally-not-known assessment measures in the tongue and in the skin (Chapter Four). Additionally, we have given considerable attention to the association of vitamin C and oral health and sickness (Chapter Nine). Finally, we have released a number of reports on the connection between carbohydrate metabolism in general and diabetes mellitus in particular in terms of vitamin C state (Chapter Eight).

A Not-Too-Much-Talked-About Medical Secret

There are obvious serious illnesses. We'll be dealing with some of these at more appropriate times later. It is also clear that there are obvious not-so-important problems. What is generally ignored are the no-so-obvious serious signals. A case in point is generally described as bruising, black and blue marks, easy injuries and poor healing. Variations of this same problem are described as varicose veins, varicosity, spider webs and even hemorrhoids. However tagged by the public, in medical lingo they are labeled as **petechia**, **ecchymosis**, **purpura**. Medically it spells poor **capillary** health.

Capillary well-being is measureable. Early in the century the Hess Test was developed. It is also referred to as the Rumpel-Leede procedure, the tourniquet test, and the negative suction technique. In all of these, blood to the arm is partially interrupted for a set period of minutes. Following the release of pressure, the number of **petechae** are counted.

T.P. Eddy from the Department of Human Nutrition at the London School of Hygiene and Tropical Medicine has reviewed and analyzed earlier work done with capillary resistance.[9] In one report, 80 elderly hospital patients were studied. Forty were given a daily multivitamin tablet containing 200 mg ascorbic acid for a year and 40 controls were provided a placebo. Measurements of leucocyte ascorbic acid were made at three-monthly intervals. The Hess test for measuring capillary strength was performed at these same times. In general, there is evidence that the capillary strength patterns paralleled the vitamin C concentration. In other words, the better (higher) the blood vitamin C state, the fewer the small hemorrhages in the skin.

The Now and New Scurvy

We have seen vitamin C's effect on scurvy. We will learn (Chapter Five) that what makes vitamin C so wonderful is its versatility. One of its roles is the improvement in capillary health. Hence, there is another way of looking at the problem. Any clinical disorder characterized by poor capillary state may be viewed as potentially one more evidence of the new and now scurvy.

So, how does this all tie together?

Mark Schultz from the Hospital of the Rockefeller Institute for Medical Research in New York, way back in 1936, studied 56 patients, aged 4 to 19 years, each of whom had experienced one or more attacks of rheumatic fever in previous years and was presently nonhospitalized.[10] Of these, 28 were assigned to Group A and received ascorbic acid (100 mg daily by mouth);

28 carefully matched patients constituted Group B and were administered lactose placebo capsules. Capillary **fragility** showed a decrease in the mean vascular health of the control group from January to April. This is simply another way of indicating a worsening in blood vessel integrity. During the same time, the average strength of the supplemented group increased. Hence, there was improvement in vascular function. It would seem that many of these patients with quiescent rheumatic fever had indeed subclinical ascorbic acid deficiency. On the other hand, Group A appeared to be partially protected from this by the ascorbic acid supplement. However, this ascorbate dose (100 mg daily) didn't prevent recurrence of rheumatic activity.

If indeed vascular resistance is a component of rheumatic fever and if it can be modified by ascorbate, then there is a suggestion of a real connection between **hypovitamin** C and the rheumatic fever state.

Summary and Conclusions

The original vitamin C connection was discovered eons ago with the recognition that an absence of vitamin C led to a fatal disease known as scurvy. When the connection was finally and firmly established, the scientific community rested with the happy thought that here was a specific vitamin associated with a specific syndrome. The tie seemed so neat and clean that one couldn't conceive that the bond was only the tip of the proverbial iceberg. While the initial relationship was identified years ago, the notion of a bigger and better connection is relatively new.

And so, *Vitamin C . . . who needs it?* To the extent that one can hazard a guess at this early point in our discussion . . . everybody who has a problem. This makes the story even more exciting since, in the last chapter, we discovered that even those without problems may well be favorably influenced!

3

THE PARTY LINE: RDAs ... AND BEYOND

Dietary assessment is not new. The earliest medical writings confirm that estimates of eating habits, albeit recorded in primitive style, have been around for a long time. Even in this day and age of technologic wonders, the dietary diary constitutes the most common method of measuring food and drink intake. True, there have been refinements. We now can look at approximately 40 different nutrients made possible by seven, four, three or one-day records as well as through computerized food frequency questionnaires. Also, there are now more sophisticated food composition tables that provide the number of milligrams of vitamin X or micrograms of mineral Y. But, for our purposes here, what is important is that more often than not, the appraisal of what one eats and drinks is still relatively crude. For more particulars regarding current methodology and philosophy, it might be well to turn to Doctor James

Levine and his colleague at the Academic Department of Medicine, The Royal Free Hospital and School of Medicine in London.[1]

In all fairness, the most sophisticated current evaluation is possible by placing a subject in a metabolic ward and measuring intake and output under hi-tech (unfortunately expensive) conditions. However, most importantly, it's not how many milligrams of this or micrograms of that but what does it all mean in terms of the adequacy of our diet? In any case, the bottom line is, "Are our eating habits (and especially vitamin C) inviting health or sickness?"

With increasing interest in diet/nutrition and with the spiraling new information becoming available, the scientific community began to make attempts in the late 1930s to design recommendations for the major foodstuffs as well as the quantity of each vitamin and mineral necessary in the daily diet. The League of Nations, the predecessor of the United Nations (UN), appointed a blue-ribbon committee to create a set of international standards. In fact, they actually were commissioned to define "the principles of nutrition best suited to ensure the fullest development and the maintenance of the organism." It was concluded "the adult's requirement (for vitamin C) is no doubt covered by about 30 mgs daily, which has been shown to be a curative dose for adults suffering from scurvy." These standards were to become a factor in important decisions to be made in Britain from 1939 on, with the outbreak of World War II.

Compared to What?

The first edition of the U.S. Recommended Dietary

Allowances (RDAs) was published in 1943 during World War II with the objective of "providing standards to serve as a goal for good nutrition." (It might be well to note that the original RDA was 75 mg of vitamin C for an adult.) In subsequent editions, the point was made that:

> . . . the recommendations are not requirements, since they represent, not merely minimal needs of average persons, but nutrient levels selected to cover individual variations in a substantial majority of the population and . . . to provide the increased needs in times of stress . . .

In the last edition (Tenth),[2] the RDAs are defined as follows:

> . . . the levels of intake of essential nutrients that, on the basis of scientific knowledge, are judged by the Food and Nutrition Board to be adequate to meet the known nutrient needs of practically all healthy persons . . .

Hence, in plain and simple language, it should be emphasized that the RDAs are intended to satisfy the health needs of healthy individuals. The sticky point is that nowhere in the Tenth Revised Edition is health defined!

For us, what does this mean in terms of vitamin C? In general, the Subcommittee has offered few changes from its last suggestions in 1985. It proposes that 60 mg continue to be the accepted, for both adult male and female, recommendation.

How possible is this to achieve?

To satisfy the current 60 mg per day vitamin C requirement means eating approximately three servings of fresh vegetables and two fresh fruits daily. According to the best available evidence today from the National Institutes of Health[3] only 9% of Americans are in optimal vitamin C state.

The single most significant change by the Subcommittee is that "regular smokers ingest at least 100 mg of vitamin C daily." This information has been known since approximately 1940. In fact, Pelletier[4] emphasized this point in a presentation at the 53rd Annual Meeting of the Federation of American Societies of Experimental Biology in Atlantic City in April 1969.

Lighting Up

In the mid-60s, well-documented statements about tobacco and vitamin C appeared. For example, one cigarette destroyed at least 25 mg of C in the body. Also, smokers of 20 cigarettes or more per day did not excrete any ascorbic acid in the urine. These remarks were being used to promote the usage of large doses of vitamin C by smokers supposedly deficient in this vitamin. On the basis of the current recommendations, two objective studies are reported.[5] The first comprises five smokers and five non-smokers, and the second 14 smokers and 14 nonsmokers.

Schectman and his cohorts posed some fascinating questions at the National Meeting of the American Federation for Clinical Research in Washington, D.C., in May 1990.[6] These Medical College of Wisconsin investigators asked, "Is 100 mgs of vitamin C enough to protect against the smoking habit?" To answer this question, they examined the records of 11,582 adult respondents in the National Health and Nutrition

Examination Survey (NHANES). **Serum AA** concentrations and the risk of low vitamin C levels for smokers consuming different amounts of the ascorbates were compared with those for nonsmokers whose ascorbic acid intake exceeded the RDA of 60 mg. Serum AA concentrations were reduced, and risk of low vitamin C increased, in smokers maintaining ascorbic acid intakes greater than 60, 100 and 150 mg. Only smokers consuming more than 200 mgs of AA per day had serum ascorbate concentrations and risk of low vitamin C equivalent to nonsmokers meeting the RDA.

The subject of tobacco consumption in particular and the bigger topic of social habits (e.g. alcohol, laxative use, contraceptive pills) as they relate to vitamin C state will receive further attention (Chapter Fifteen).

Reading the RDA Another Way

Thus far we have provided the vitamin C description that will protect us against the worst situation, namely scurvy. We shall learn (Chapter Five) that ascorbic acid serves many vital and wonderful roles. One must wonder what would be the desired vitamin C requirement to deal with any one or any combination of the functions known to be associated with optimal ascorbate state.

Emil Ginter from the Research Institute of Human Nutrition in Czechoslovakia[7] raises the interesting point:

> Ideal RDA should be based on studies with increasing vitamin C doses in which the efficiency of the ascorbate-dependent systems would be correlated with the vitamin C concentration in the target tissues . . .

In other words, "how much vitamin C is necessary to maintain the 'ideal' serum cholesterol concentration?" In his own words:

> It is probable that in healthy adults, such a dose ranges from 100 to 200 mg and that in stress conditions, it exceeds 200 mg per day.

Here again is another challenge to the party line!

Is there still another way of ascertaining the amount of vitamin C necessary to maintain health in healthy subjects? We think so.

At the University Medical Center in Birmingham, our group got involved a number of years ago in the health of members of the health profession.

Using 1038 dentists and their spouses as subjects we calculated daily reported vitamin C consumption from an (admittedly crude) food frequency questionnaire.[8-9] This form assessed the C consumed from both diet and ascorbic acid or multivitamin supplementation. Clinical state was graded by the Cornell Medical Health Questionnaire (CMI). The CMI is a self-administered health questionnaire consisting of 195 queries. Respondents answer each question by circling the word "yes" or "no." Each interrogative is phrased so that the affirmative answers indicate **pathology**. The clinical findings in this report are the total number of positive CMI responses (score).

Line 1 (Table 3.1) shows the daily vitamin C consumption of the entire group of doctors and their spouses. In this sample of 1038, the CMI ranged from 0 to 125 with a mean of 16. The daily reported vitamin C intake spread from 15 to 1120 mg. Imagine, there are allegedly healthy doctors consuming only 25% (15 mg) of the RDA! The average ascorbic acid was 327 mg per day. This, incidentally, is five or sixfold more than the RDA. (Both the American Medical Association (AMA) and the American Dental Association (ADA) have indicated that the type of doctor interested in his or her own health and willing to be studied as in this survey is already above average in health.) Hence, in the usual context, these values would be viewed as "ideal" when, in fact, they are only normal (average).

Table 3.1

The "ideal" vitamin C intake					
	Sample Size	CMI Range	Mean	Vitamin C (mg) Range	Mean
total sample	1038	0-125	15.9	15-1120	327
<CMI 30	912	0-29	12.4	41-1120	335
<CMI 15	581	0-14	7.9	41-1120	349
<CMI 5	113	0-4	2.8	49-1120	376
<CMI 4	73	0-3	2.1	104-736	383
<CMI 3	46	0-2	1.5	108-736	389
<CMI 2	16	0-1	0.6	116-719	390
<CMI 0	6	0	0.0	120-719	410

Deleting all subjects with 30 or more symptoms and signs leaves a sample of 912 (line 2), a clinical mean of 12, a vitamin C range of 41-1120 mg, and an average of 335 mg per day. Proceeding through the eight lines of this chart, the daily vitamin C intake slowly and systematically rises as the number of allowable clinical symptomatology (CMI score) is reduced. This approach indicates that the clinically healthier the sample, the greater the daily vitamin C intake. Under the conditions of this experiment, approximately 410 mg of vitamin C may be designated as the acceptable daily allowance for healthy people who wish to maintain health. This is about seven times the RDA!

A Mind-Boggling Addendum

It is well to reexamine our last experiment. It was performed on modern people and reported in 1977. It's an inexpensive and simple and more importantly a common sense approach to the problem. As far as we know, it has never been confirmed or disavowed . . . until now.

We discover that two prominent paleontologists, Eaton and Konner from Atlanta, in their magnificent and monumental report,[10] outline the diet of our remote ancestors as a reference standard for modern human nutrition and a model for defense against certain so-called diseases of civilization.

Apropos vitamin C, they estimate from the mean ascorbic acid content of 27 vegetables consumed by hunter-gatherers that the average vitamin C intake would have been 392.3 mg per day in paleolithic diets.

Imagine, Eaton and Konner (from their sophisticated and elaborate study of primitive man) come up with 392 mg; from our investigation of modern man, we find 410 mg, a matter of 4% difference!

And there's more. We shall discover (Chapter Eleven) that men consuming 300 to 400 mg of vitamin C daily tend to live approximately six years longer!

Serendipity . . . or confirmation?!?

Can We Do Better?

Thus far, we have two different answers to the ascorbate requirement based on two separate definitions of hypovitaminosis C. First, the official RDA is 60 mg and will protect against the classical hypovitaminosis C state, namely scurvy. Second, we've been studying the RDA from another vantage point based upon the hypothesis that relatively symptomless and sign-free persons are healthier than those with clinical symptomatology. By this approach, the RDA should be about 400 mg per day . . . a matter of almost seven times the traditional RDA.

While the RDA may be used as a crude measure of acceptability, the Optimal Recommended Dietary Allowance (ORDA) or IRDA ("Ideal" Recommended Dietary Allowance) is suggested as a more sophisticated approach to vitamin C in health and disease. Here we wish to emphasize the ultimate, the most sophisticated, the most theoretical level. This would represent, as it were, the custom-built prescription for an individual. It would not only recognize the importance of tobacco consumption earlier mentioned but the effects of drugs such as aspirin, the contraceptive pill, laxatives, and other conditions as they influence vitamin C state (Chapter Fifteen).

Summary and Conclusions

And so, *Vitamin C . . . who needs it?*

From a dietary/nutritional standpoint, there are actually four answers.

First, if you are **scorbutic** or fearful of it and wish to protect yourself against it, then the answer is simple, clear, and available. The Food and Nutrition Board of the National Nutritional Council in its Tenth Revised edition assures us that one requires only about 10 to 20 mgs of vitamin C. Hence, their recommendation of 60 mgs per day guarantees that there will be no evidence of classical scurvy.

How much does one need to simply remain in so-called good health? The RDA is still 60 mgs. However, viewing the body by other methodologies challenges the RDA. If one asks how much is needed to discourage **hypercholesterolemia** then the RDA should be of an order of 200 or more mgs of ascorbate per day. This is roughly three or four times the traditional recommendation. If one views the problem in a symptomless and sign-free format, then the RDA should be about seven-fold.

We have learned that, for the first time, the Food and Nutrition Board has recognized a different need under one social condition (tobacco consumption). We have also discovered that the RDA for smokers may be too low. It is safe to conclude that further revision of the RDA will probably deal with other social factors (e.g. alcohol, laxative use, contraceptive pills, drugs).

Finally, what we would really like to discover — beyond the RDA — is the Ideal or Optimal Recommended Dietary Allowances (IRDA or ORDA). This subject will be examined very carefully in subsequent chapters.

For the moment, it must be emphasized that arriving at sober estimates by dietary means is difficult if not impossible. Can one reach a better estimate of optimal vitamin C state by other techniques? To do this, the next chapter will consider the subject as biochemical briefs.

4

BIOCHEMICAL
SNAPSHOTS

It is no great feat to make a diagnosis of scurvy when a patient presents the classical symptomatology. It's even easier to confirm the suspicion when the victim obviously is consuming a vitamin C free diet. This was the usual sequence of events in days past. Even in this day and age, one occasionally meets up with the classical picture. However, more often than not, the clinical story isn't so sharply defined and is further complicated by a fuzzy dietary record. Not infrequently it's no longer a simple matter to establish a scorbutic diagnosis.

It helps to have help. Fortunately, there are some obvious and not-so-obvious biochemical tools available which make it possible to match up the more subtle clinical picture and the questionable dietary pattern. From a practical standpoint, only a few such tests are available. These serve as a subject for discussion in this chapter.

By Popular Demand . . . The Plasma Ascorbic Acid Concentration

The vitamin C levels in the blood and in some of its components have been studied for quite some time. Plasma ascorbic acid is presently the most popular test. The technique has been extensively described and the procedure is simple and relatively inexpensive.

There are two principal shortcomings. First, plasma ascorbic acid is more a function of dietary intake than tissue state. Second, it is still not clear as to what constitutes the normal range and even less the ideal state.

The Interdepartmental Committee on Nutrition for National Defense (ICNND) has expended considerable attention to plasma levels since early in the 1940s. Originally, they declared that any plasma level below 0.1 mg% should be viewed as suboptimal. During the next decade or so they changed their minds with rising recommendations of 0.2, 0.4 and 0.6 mg%. You will find, laced throughout this book, that many if not most of the experts utilize 0.4 to 0.6 mg% to define acceptable levels. However, there are those who will argue for much higher optimal values.

Emil Ginter made the point (Chapter Three) that perhaps a better way of establishing vitamin C norms is by examining its relationship to known metabolic functions. In this regard, Buzina and his colleagues in Zagreb[1] studied vitamin C and the oral cavity. Their comments:

> The 4-hydroxyproline and proline content of peri-dontal tissue was measured in 24 adult volunteers

with initially low and partially even deficient plasma vitamin C values, before and after peroral supplementation with 70 mg of ascorbic acid daily for six weeks . . . There was a statistically significant rise and normalization respectively of plasma ascorbic acid and simultaneously a statistically significant increase of the hydroxyproline and proline in peridontal tissue but not before the plasma vitamin C level was above 0.9 mg/dl. The optimal plasma vitamin C level which was associated with the highest hydroxyproline and proline content in periodontal tissue ranged between 1.00-1.30 mg/dl corresponding to the total dietary ascorbic acid intake of about 100 mg.

We'll mention **hydroxylation** later (Chapter Five). Also, we'll return to the ascorbates in **stomatology** (Chapter Nine). For the moment, the point being made is that it may well be that 1.0 mg% is the preferred plasma vitamin C concentration. This view is held by others.[2] It's at variance though with current thinking.[3] What's critical is that where one draws the line dictates the frequency of hypoascorbemia.

An Alternative . . . The Buffy Coat Vitamin C Layer

As we have noted, there is still confusion regarding the standards for plasma vitamin C concentration. The other big objection is the consensus that plasma ascorbic acid is more a measure of dietary intake than tissue concentration.

In recent times, efforts have been made to quantify the concentration of vitamin C in a readily available tissue, namely blood. There are today so-called norms for ascorbic acid in **leukocytes, erythrocytes,** and platelets. The most popular of these tests consist of the measurement of vitamin C in the **buffy coat layer** (which includes all of these cellular elements). "Normal" is somewhere between 25.0 and 38.0 mcgs/10^8. (Incidentally, this is another way of expressing the density of vitamin C per one hundred million cells.) Once again, there are considerable differences of opinion as to the desired values in health versus sickness.

The burning question is how many people, by this method, show suboptimal vitamin C state? C. J.

Table 4.1

percentage of population groups with unequivocally low leukocyte vitamin C reserves	
group	**percentage of subjects with classical scurvy**
young, healthy	0
elderly, healthy	3
elderly, outpatients	20
institutionalized young	30
patients with cancer	46
institutionalized elderly	50

Schorah provides us with some exciting answers.[4] Table 4.1 summarizes the approximate frequency of classical scurvy in different samples as judged by the buffy coat layer. It is obvious that somewhere between zero percent of healthy young subjects to one out of two institutionalized elderly may possibly demonstrate biochemically full-blown classical scurvy. With regard to

the shades-of-grey (Table 4.2), the evidence suggests
that somewhere between three percent of young and

Table 4.2

percentage of population groups with marginal leukocyte vitamin C reserves	
group	percentage of subjects with marginal Vitamin C deficiency state
young, healthy	3
elderly, healthy	20
elderly, outpatients	68
patients with cancer	76
institutionalized elderly	95
institutionalized young	100

healthy subjects and 100 percent of institutionalized
young suffer from marginal hypovitaminosis C.
Whatever the figures, what seems unquestioned is that
a significant segment of the population shows biochemical evidence of vitamin C deficiency! This is a good
time to reflect on the patient/doctor conversation
described earlier (Chapter One).

While the buffy coat layer is viewed at present as
the best test, it is not without its problems. For one, it
isn't readily available. Additionally, it is a technically
difficult and costly procedure. Finally, as has already
been mentioned, there is still some question as to the
normal/ideal range. For these and other reasons, it is
not surprising that there's a continued interest in
other, hopefully more readily available and simpler, tissue measures of ascorbate state.

How Deep is the Skin (Vitamin C)?

Now enter the University of Alabama Medical Center . . .

The so-called **intradermal** ascorbic acid test was originally designed (in the 1930s) to ascertain, in a quick and relatively simple fashion, a reasonable **integumentary** measure of vitamin C state. An extensive analysis of its history and findings, in both lower animals and humans, has been described in two earlier reports.[5,6] As a matter of fact, you may recall (Chapter One), this is how we originally got involved.

Without pursuing the specifics, which have already been published, the test consists of an intradermal injection of a 2, 6-dichlorphenolindophenol (blue) dye. The results (expressed in minutes) are based on the disappearance of the blue color. The shorter time required for decolorization, the higher the vitamin C density in the skin. Conversely, the longer the vanishing time, the poorer the vitamin C concentration. A generally acceptable ascorbic acid grade is approximately 10 to 15 minutes. A poor vitamin C condition shows up in a test which extends up to one hour.

The intradermal test has been compared to other procedures and especially to the plasma ascorbic acid concentration. Figure 4.1 is designed to demonstrate the plasma ascorbate level in a group of 16 presumably healthy dental students before (under fasting conditions) and at set times after the intravenous injection of 1000 mgs of vitamin C.[7] Note that the initial C level was 0.5 mg%. Within 15 minutes, the ascorbate concentration rose to 1.3 (an increase of 140%). Twenty four and 48 hours later, plasma levels were still considerably higher than originally.

There are several points worth emphasis. If indeed 1.0 mg% appears to be the acceptable vitamin C plas-

Figure 4.1

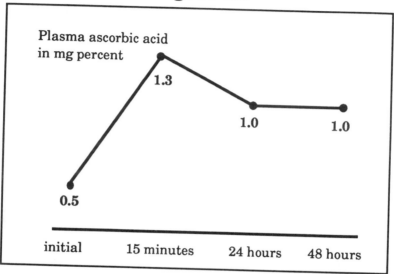

Plasma ascorbic acid in mg percent

1.3

1.0   1.0

0.5

initial   15 minutes   24 hours   48 hours

ma score, then these presumably healthy dental students are hardly healthy with a fasting 0.5 value. It is also noteworthy that this single jolt of vitamin C by vein elicits a 24 to 48 hour after-effect.

Additionally, in these same students and at the very same time, the intradermal test was performed. Figure 4.2 summarizes these findings. The initial (fasting) preinjection time was 24 minutes. The time decreased to 12 (in effect dropped 50%) and returned slowly to almost the original levels within 48 hours.

There are a number of items to be underlined. First, the initial intradermal time is 24 minutes. You may recall that the so-called normal range is 15 to 25 minutes. Hence, we note here a marginal vitamin C state as judged in the skin. Secondly, it's exciting to note how much and how quickly the vitamin C reaches the skin. Third, within 24 to 48 hours, the original values are restored. Fourth and most importantly, the pictures for the skin and those earlier for plasma are mirror images. Finally, it is fair to conclude that, whatever the benefits of plasma determinations are, they are possible with this not-so-well-known procedure.

Figure 4.2

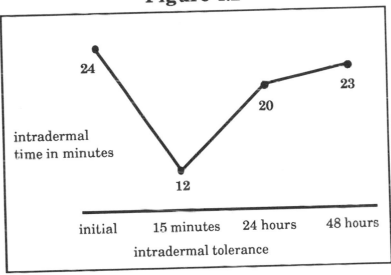

The Mouth ... A Unique Vitamin C Testing Site

An even more readily available and simple procedure has been provided to us by Giza and his group in Poland in the 1960s. The technique is very simple and has been described by us in a number of publications.

One drop of a 1/340 N 2, 6-dicholoroindophenol sodium salt solution is deposited on the **dorsum** of the tongue. Just as the drop lands, timing is initiated with a stopwatch and is continued until the blue color has disappeared. This test only takes seconds.

The **Lingual Ascorbic Acid Test** (usually abbreviated LAAT) time of approximately 20 seconds or less indicates that the tissue is well-supplied with ascorbic acid; 20 to 25 seconds reflects a marginal or suboptimal vitamin C tissue level; and greater than 25 seconds indicates a definite ascorbate deficit.

What have we found? Depending upon the standards for normality and ideality, it has been concluded that somewhere between 17 and 72 percent of the subjects studied by us demonstrated suboptimal to clearcut ascorbic acid deficiency levels. So, *Vitamin C . . . who needs it?* Utilizing this simple tongue test, just about everybody would fare better in some way.

We provided earlier some respectability to the intradermal test time by comparing it with the generally-approved plasma ascorbic acid level. What happens when such an analysis is made with the tongue test?

The relationship of the fasting and non-fasting Lingual Vitamin C Test scores and plasma ascorbic acid concentration was studied in 1194 subjects.[8] The evidence suggests that there is a significant negative correlation between these two test procedures. In other words, the higher (better) the plasma level, the lower (shorter or better) the lingual time.

It is abundantly clear (Figure 4.3) within the limits of this study that there is a significant mirror-image connection between lingual test time scores and plasma ascorbic acid levels under fasting conditions.

We even have a fairly clear notion of what constitutes the ideal Lingual Vitamin C Test time through a study of presumably healthy young men.[9] This was accomplished by a selection on the basis of rigid health criteria. Individuals with symptoms and signs of disease were progressively eliminated. The technique has been described earlier (Chapter Three). The evidence, within the limits of this investigation, suggests that the physiologic range for the lingual vitamin C test may be quite restricted, approximately 15 to 25 seconds.

Figure 4.3

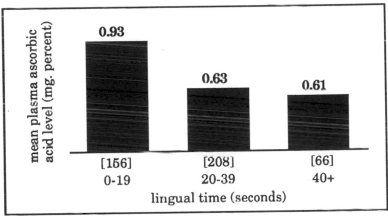

There are many other interesting and exciting bits of information about the tongue test. To provide the reader with some measure of the sensitivity of the lingual test, the scores, under fasting conditions, were studied three weeks apart in subjects receiving placebo versus C (100 mg three times daily) supplementation.[10] It is abundantly clear that a statistically significant reduction in lingual time occurred only in the ascorbic acid supplemented group.

What else do we know about these rarely discussed biochemical snapshots?

Six hundred and sixteen subjects participated in a study designed to examine the relationship of the lingual vitamin C test scores and intradermal vitamin C test times.[11] The evidence from the entire sample suggests that there is a statistically convincing positive correlation. In other words, the longer the lingual test (in seconds), the longer the intradermal time (in minutes). The limited evidence present suggests that the relationship between fasting intradermal and lingual time is higher than the correlation of lingual time and plasma ascorbic acid.

In general, we have learned that the lingual test, while not the most sophisticated procedure, can serve the clinician successfully. Literally hundreds if not thousands of practitioners use the test in their office environments. Rarely have there been publications stemming from their observations. However, Sarji, et al. of the Veterans Administration Medical Center at the University of South Carolina, has examined the platelet vitamin C levels in diabetics versus nondiabetic subjects utilizing successfully the lingual vitamin C test.[12] In the interest of completeness, there are some few researchers who have reported difficulty with the reproducibility of this procedure.[13]

Other Not-So-Obvious Biochemical Briefs

We are ready to make the bold prediction that when studied, we shall learn that every cell, and therefore every tissue, organ, and site, is vitamin C dependent.

Hence, it figures that when all the evidence is in, all diseases and conditions will be, to a varying degree, AA dependent.

By now, we have already presented some evidence to underscore this point. Many different and diverse problems, described in earlier chapters, have been shown to benefit from ascorbate supplementation under supervised experimental conditions.

We will discover (Chapter Five) that practically all major metabolic processes are connected to this extraordinary vitamin.

To further emphasize how far-reaching the implications are, we will here and now discuss common clinical problems by means of not-so-common experimental studies.

There is no question but that allergies and hypersensitivities (albeit variously defined) are frequently encountered in the general public. There is the overview estimate that approximately, on any given day, 25 million Americans are suffering with some form of allergy. While much about the hypersensitivity state is still arguable, there's one point which is unquestioned. During the allergic phenomenon, histamine is released. As a matter of fact, it is well-known, even in the public domain, that one of the most effective treatments for allergies is the use of antihistaminic agents. What is not commonly recognized is that one, if not the most powerful orthomolecular antihistamine, is vitamin C. Is there a relationship between histamine and the ascorbates?

It has been known for some time, from guinea pig studies, that when vitamin C is withdrawn, the blood histamine levels begin to rise in a matter of 72 hours.

Capitalizing on this and other information,

Clemetson, then at the Methodist Hospital in Brooklyn, New York,[14] administered oral ascorbate (one gram daily for three days) to 11 selected volunteers. The result was a reduction of the blood histamine level in every instance. A separate analysis of 437 human blood samples has shown that when the plasma ascorbic acid level falls below 1.0 mg%, the whole blood histamine level rises exponentially as the ascorbic acid level decreases. When the vitamin C level declines below 0.7 mg%, there's a highly significant increase in the blood histamine level.

Summary and Conclusions

There is no longer a need to guess the vitamin C state. There are biochemical tests. Some are more common than others; a few are more expensive. There are also less known but available simple tissue measures. Two of interest to us over many years have been the intradermal (skin) and the lingual (tongue) tests.

What is most important and relevant is, utilizing these testing procedures, *Vitamin C . . . who needs it?* By all measures available, it is clear that just about everybody demonstrates suboptimal state.

We have alluded to the versatility of vitamin C. What we've not emphasized, by means of supervised experimentation, are the reasons. In Chapter Five, we'll take a hard look at the C in panacea.

5

THERE'S A C
IN PANACEA

Right or wrong . . . good or bad . . . we live in a
bizarre world. We insist that Agent A is necessary to
solve Medical Problem A (e.g. acne). We're assured that
Factor B is the answer to Syndrome B (i.e. baldness).
This logic understandably explains why Preparation H
happily helps hemorrhoids. And so, it's not surprising,
by extension, that we believe that smoking causes lung
cancer. We're dead sure that sooner or later we'll find
the virus for arthritis and that baking in the sun
makes for skin cancer.

When a compound, call it C, seems to solve many
problems, it's tagged as snake oil. This conjures up the
state fair, the midway, the medicine show, and the han-
dle-barred mustached hawker peddling Lydia
Pinkham.

What we have not been told are all and the real
facts. The truth is that more people who smoke don't

have lung cancer than do. There are more sun-lovers without skin tumors than with. In other words, the answers to many, if not most, of our problems aren't as simple as we have been led to believe.

So, where does vitamin C fit into this story?

The Nuts and Bolts

According to the strange scientists who slave in the subatomic caves, vitamin C performs its wonderful feats because it serves as an electron donor. In other words, ascorbic acid (AA) has the extraordinary capacity to transfer tiny submicroscopic electrical particles. That seems to satisfy the superscientists but, for Mr. and Mrs. America it's a shallow explanation. What the person-on-the-street wants to know is why people feel better when these little electrons are moved around.

What makes sense to Mr. and Mrs. Public is that this microscopic activity makes possible many well-known and not-too-well-known physiochemical reactions. Even those of us who aren't scientifically trained have heard of **oxidation** and reduction, **methylation,** hydroxylation (we mentioned this in the last chapter), and **peroxidation**. Some of these we'll refer to in this very chapter; others will be emphasized later at more appropriate times and places.

But even these chemical feats are difficult to understand for the untrained. What the public would really like to know is how these physiocochemical mechanisms fit into the ecologic system and wind up making people healthier and happier.

There are many well-known physiologic events associated with ascorbate metabolism . . . too many in fact to discuss here. However, we will cite some representative examples derived from scientifically sound experiments.

The Hot and Cold Facts

It is remarkable, when one thinks about it, that we live in a world the temperature of which can change from sub-freezing to blistering heat. Notwithstanding, the human organism's thermostat remains remarkably constant. When it doesn't, there are serious consequences. One of the evidences of disturbance in thermoregulation in a practical sense is demonstrated by the large number of people who cannot tolerate even small changes in heat and cold. They are, in fact, hostages during either the winter or summer months. Here's a possible snake oil story.

For the moment, it is fascinating to note that body temperature can be significantly modified by relatively small amounts of AA and in short order under controlled conditions.

Carol S. Johnston, Ph.D., presented a report (subsequently published)[1] at the Federation of American Societies for Experimental Biology's Annual meeting in April 1969. The purpose of her study was to demonstrate ascorbate-induced hyperthermia in humans under simple and controlled conditions.

Ten healthy men and women aged 18 to 40 years were screened by personal interview for a recent history of medication, illness, drug use, tobacco, unusual dietary habits, and supplemental vitamins. The subjects reported to the test site at 8:00 A.M. in a resting and fasted state. Oral temperatures were recorded by digital thermometry at 9:00 A.M. and fasting blood samples were collected at the same time (blood vitamin

C was ascertained). Subsequently, the subjects matched by age and sex consumed either l-ascorbic acid in tablet form or an indistinguishable placebo. A double-blind protocol was utilized throughout the study. Temperature was self-recorded by each subject at one hour intervals following the blood draw. Beginning at 9:00 A.M., measurements were taken every 60 minutes for eight hours. Additionally, blood samples were collected at 4 and 24 hours post-treatment.

Several points are worthy of special mention. Mean oral body temperature was significantly elevated (0.7°F) within two hours following one gram of vitamin C. In parallel, plasma ascorbate rose 32% over the control group in the first four hours. This simple study indicates that a single oral dose of ascorbic acid at levels approximately 17 times the so-called recommended intake elevates body temperature significantly in healthy men and women.

As the investigator from Arizona State University points out, fever is commonly observed in man following exposure with infectious/inflammatory agents. It is interesting that AA administration may enhance disease resistance. Fever (the elevation of body temperature resulting from disease) is postulated to benefit the infected host by augmenting certain types of cell proliferation and by other mechanisms. This point will be elaborated on later (Chapter Six). What is important here is to underscore the fact that ascorbate is an essential ingredient in one of man's vital defense systems.

Here is an excellent example, by means of a very simple, neat, and clean experiment, showing one of the properties of vitamin C which unequivocally qualifies it as an extraordinary ecologic agent!

More About the Sticky Story

We ought not to be surprised. In Chapter One we learned that fertility is in part a function of sperm stickiness. Vitamin C tends to encourage unstickiness leading to increased sperm motility and the greater chance of conception.

The ascorbates are also vital to platelet stickiness. These little blood cells circulate constantly. They serve to plug up minor injuries. Hence, they are required in critical amounts for clotting. The flip side is that the quality and/or quantity of these platelets should be such as to discourage too much clotting. This is, in many cases, because of platelet stickiness.

Platelet health has been measured and is reported abundantly in the scientific literature. The high-falutin' formidable titles are platelet adhesiveness (PaI), platelet aggregation (PAg), platelet adhesive index (PAI), and platelet aggregation ratio (PAgR). While these terms connote different measures of platelet activity, they collectively describe the ability (or inability) of the **thrombocytes** performing one of their vital functions.

To recap . . . one of the functions of the platelets is to clump and plug minor damaged areas in blood vessels. Hence, a degree of stickiness is necessary. Obviously, situations which make the blood too sticky are undesirable. This phenomenon can be experimentally created by providing a presumably healthy subject with a small amount of butter.

Two Indian physicians provide us with an interesting story based on an unique experimental design.[2]

A. Bordia and S. K. Varma of the Department of Medicine (Cardiology) and Indigenous Drug Research Centre in Tagore at the Medical College and Hospital studied the effect of oral administration of ascorbic acid on PAI, PAgR, and serum vitamin C levels. These investigators provided ten presumably healthy male subjects with 75 grams of butter. Would you believe that this enhanced the tendency of platelet clumping at the end of only four hours? But, by adding one gram of ascorbic acid supplementation with the fatty meal, the **agglutination** was distinctly minimized.

What really does all this mean? Can one conclude that butter is bad? Does this experiment confirm that butter invites platelet stickiness? Is this the whole story? Might it not be that low ascorbate levels are the real reason for the exaggerated agglutination? None of these queries are answered in the Bordia experiment. What we know for sure is that a more **physiologic platelet** state can be obtained with AA supplementation under these conditions.

They also studied sick people. Specifically, they investigated 20 patients with coronary artery disease (CAD) under double-blind conditions. One group was provided with vitamin C for ten days at a dose of one gram every eight hours and demonstrated that the PAg was significantly improved. Coincidentally, this was paralleled by a rise in plasma vitamin C concentration.

What is striking here is that such studies emphasize a unique property of the ascorbates in both sick and healthy people. It may be of considerable importance in the prevention and treatment of chronic **thromboatherosclerotic** disease. This is by no means the end—we will return to these Indian Researchers in Chapter Seven.

Fire Quenchers

Throughout the ages, attempts have been made to explain health and sickness. All have contained a modicum of truth and a lot of fancy. Now we have a theory of health/sickness which is a distillation of all that has transpired based on more and new evidence and derived from more and new sophisticated instrumentation.

In the now and new twentieth century hypothesis, it is clear that specific agents for specific diseases are a woefully lacking and incomplete theory. In this day and age, more and more people are beginning to recognize that the phenomenon is multifactorial. Phrased in simple arithmetic language, how well we fare or sick we get depends upon a whole series of challenges and our ability to cope with these many and different bombardments.

More revolutionary is the fact that this hostile world is made up of a multiplex of noxious agents. What is especially exciting is that these universal clobberings eventuate in universal diseases. In other words, as wild as it may seem, these very same challenges contribute to seemingly different syndromes like heart disease, cancer and arthritis. In fact, there are actually published lists which confirm these relationships.[3]

What is rapidly becoming evident is that not all environmental threats need necessarily derive from the external world. **Endogenous** factors contribute devastating perturbations to the organism. For example, it is now clear that some of our blessings may indeed be double-edged and, in fact, serve as curses.

We obviously need oxygen. However, with too much or when mismanaged, there can be oxidative damage. As a matter of fact, we even now know the jawbreaking labels for some of these elements such as **theobarbituric acid reactive substances** (TBARS).[4]

It has long been appreciated, even in the earliest medical writings, that health is associated with equilibrium, balance, homeostasis, collectively tagged as harmony. On the other hand, disease spells chaos and crisis. This can be expressed in clinical, physiologic, biochemical, and even electrical terms. In this regard, the new thinking recognizes that molecules and atoms with unpaired electrical charges act irresponsibly like raucous renegades and produce molecular mayhem. In some circles, they are now called free radicals. The sequence of events eventuates in combustion, and in the minds of some experts can be likened to fire which leads to visible debris and ashes.

The good news is that there are solutions to this oxidative damage, generally called scavengers. They form a class of substances, largely nutrients, called antioxidants.

Where does vitamin C fit? In a remarkable paper by Frei and others[5] ascorbic acid is viewed as the single most important antidote or, to pursue the analogy, fire quencher.

How can this be best portrayed to the layman? Cut an apple in half. Sprinkle lemon juice (or some crystals of vitamin C) on one cut side and leave the other untouched. Watch the apple. In just a very few moments you will note spoilage (as evidenced by browning) on the nonsprinkled side. Here is a simple and clean demonstration of the unfavorable influence of oxidative damage upon an apple. Here's also an excellent demonstration of the protective effect of vitamin C.

But, what does all this mean in practical terms?

Part of the answer is in those earlier Ames studies (Chapter One). However, in the interest of completeness, the California group[6] followed ten men kept on closely monitored diets at the research center in Presidio in San Francisco. Their basic diet was devoid of fruits and vegetables, consisting primarily of protein and carbohydrates. The diet was then fortified with varying amounts of vitamin C.

At first the men received 250 mgs of ascorbic acid per day and the degree of sperm damage was noted. AA supplements were then discontinued. Thus, the subjects were receiving a mere 5 mg/day in their diets. This netted more obvious oxidative damage to the sperm. The story ends happily when vitamin C was restored to the original 250 mgs on a daily basis.

All of this recognizes the results of early chromosomal damage. There's the bigger picture of such cellular mutation later in life expressed in **carcinomatosis** and heart disease. These manifestations of genetic injury will be a later theme (Chapter Seven).

Poisons . . . Poisons . . . Everywhere

The electronic and print media explode almost daily with the not-so-good-news about pollution. Less known, at least to the public, is the fact that the exposure to many industrial products creates chromosomal damage, possible cellular mutation, and an increased carcinogenic potential. We have already learned about this possibility (Chapter One and earlier in this section).

An innovative and highly revealing demonstration comes to us from Prague. R. J. Sram and his colleagues[7] studied the possible **antimutagenic** (a fancy word for damage) potential of **prophylactically** administered AA preparations. This was conducted in a group of 35 coal-tar workers occupationally exposed to benzene products. The effectiveness of ascorbic acid prophylaxis was assessed. Workers under these conditions ordinarily show about 5% of their cells to be abnormal. These exposed workers were examined before and after a three-month treatment period with C at the daily dose of one gram for five days per week. In the exposed group, the **cytogenetic** analysis of peripheral blood lymphocytes revealed a significant (and favorable) reduction in the frequency of abberent cells from the customary 5% down to 2%. In other words, two out of three of these workers showed cellular improvement. What makes this all even more exciting is that in a group of matching controls, the frequency of abnormal cells, for practical purposes, didn't change.

The bigger picture now is that ascorbic acid markedly affects the toxic and cancer-causing properties of more than fifty different common pollutants in our air, water, and food.

Here's one more evidence of the wonders of C!

The Great Healer

Collagen is the human organism's principal protein. It's part of all tissues and therefore is critical in ligaments, tendons, blood vessels, muscle, etc.

An interesting case in point. Ascorbic acid stores are frequently depleted in paraplegic patients with pressure-sores. Vitamin C therapy may encourage collagen formation in these sores.

Here's the work of T. V. Taylor and his associates at the Manchester Royal Infirmary and University Hospital of South Manchester.[8] In a prospective double-blind controlled trial, the effect of relatively modest doses of ascorbic acid (500 mg/twice daily) on the healing of pressure-sores was assessed. Twenty surgical patients were carefully studied, the pressure areas being meticulously analyzed by serial photography and even ulcer tracings. In the group supplemented with AA, there was an average reduction in pressure-sore area of 84% after one month compared with 43% in the placebo subset. These statistically significant findings convincingly confirm that the ascorbates accelerate the health of pressure-sores.

Etcetera ... Etcetera ... Etcetera ...

It is difficult, if not impossible, to provide a complete inventory of the functions of vitamin C. For one, not all of them are yet known. Among those that are, they are variously and overlappingly classified (e.g. clinical, chemical, physiologic, and immunologic). We have already learned (Chapter One) that ascorbic acid can contribute to statural change. This can be viewed as a clinical benefit. On the other hand, the mechanism by which height is altered is generally ascribed to collagen synthesis. This same phenomenon can also be credited in the chemical column.

There are many exciting summarizations that all suggest the multiplex of functions. For example, *Nutrition Reviews*[9] emphasizes the well-known point that vitamin C enhances the absorption of iron. It also underscores the fact that the ascorbates play a significant role in the utilization and assimilation of other metals.

The story goes on . . . we will soon discover many other roles for C.

Summary and Conclusions

We made the point earlier that every cell, and consequently all tissues, organs, and sites, are vitamin C dependent. Representative intermediary processes have been discussed. Documentation from simple double-blind studies is provided to emphasize the many and varied actions by which vitamin C makes for health and, under abnormal conditions, invites illness.

Now, let's turn to a survey of our leading killing and crippling problems. The emphasis, beginning with the next chapter, will be on the preventative and therapeutic role of ascorbic acid. Specifically, we will first turn our attention to the place of vitamin C in so-called infection maladies.

6

HOW NOT
TO BE BUGGED

We are now embarking on a different tack. With this chapter, we will begin a hard look at the many different faces of clinical scurvy. Infections warrant our attention because they are common problems. According to communicable disease experts, in a recent studied year, there were for every 100 inhabitants of the United States, 46 common colds, 43 influenza-like ailments, and 25 other infectious syndromes.

You may recall that the vitamin C wakeup call began with the experiences of Professor Linus Pauling and his personal encounters with the common cold. The serendipity didn't end there.

The late Professor Sherry Lewin, of the Department of Molecular Biology at London Polytechnic was plagued (as he tells it) by frequent and severe colds. He had taken to swallowing 50 mg of C each day mostly "to please my wife." One day Mrs. Lewin returned home with the only dosage she'd been able to buy . . . one gram in an effervescent tablet. Not wishing to waste the tablets (or argue with his spouse), Doctor Lewin began taking them and lo and behold he noted that the "incidence, severity, and duration" of his bad colds were greatly reduced with two or three one-gram doses each day.

Trading on his reputation as a distinguished researcher, Lewin got 69 of his cold-plagued colleagues to test vitamin C. Significant relief came to 64, a better than 90% improvement rate!

Convinced he was onto something important, Lewin undertook a long and intensive search which culminated in a book entitled *Vitamin C: Its Molecular Biology and Medical Potential.*[1]

From this chance finding have flowed many interesting epidemiologic and cause-and-effect studies regarding the ascorbates in the prevention and treatment of the common cold and other respiratory findings. Obviously, with our time and space constraints, it is our purpose here only to provide representative experiments.

The "Soil" Concept

In primitive times, people considered health and disease to be evidence of the capricious nature of the gods. They believed themselves to be cursed by illness or blessed with health, depending at all times on their relationship with the reigning deities.

A more sophisticated hypothesis evolved. The body's own internal structure was somehow linked with the onset of illness. There followed years of relentless probing for the underlying cause of disease. As late as the middle 1800s, it was generally accepted that most illnesses resulted from a disturbance in a person's internal environment.

In 1865, Louis Pasteur made a discovery from which developed the "germ theory," which dominates medicine to this day. Once people knew that formerly unheard of microorganisms could invade the body and flourish, the search to seek out, identify, and combat these environmental villains took off. Sadly, it has by no means ended.

The germ theory has suited our human ego quite well. Most of us prefer to believe that the illnesses we suffer are the result of external forces—just as we would rather blame bad luck for our failures. And so, we continually say that we "catch" a cold, "get" the flu, and "come down with" pneumonia as though we are in no way to blame for the medical catastrophe that befalls us.

Germ-theory advocates would have us view the body as a helpless quarry eternally trying to elude a multitude of disease-bearing bugs vigilantly intent upon infecting the host.

A small cadre of medical practitioners, however, has resisted the germ theory as the one sole answer to illness. They have carefully noted that while microorganisms are obviously involved in many ailments, their mere presence does not automatically guarantee disease.

Three healthy people, for example, can breathe the same germs at the same moment. One may develop pneumonia, another sniffle her way through a cold, and the third goes unscathed. After all, in the case of most epidemics, those people who succumb represent only a fraction of the number of people exposed.

Is the germ theory obsolete? More than one noted scientist now espouses a more sophisticated approach to illness. We are convinced that every disease, physical and mental, is generated by the interplay of internal and external circumstances. It logically follows that disease may be prevented or cured by correcting any of the existing variables. Obviously, we can therefore go after the "germ," and/or modify the internal milieu.

And where does vitamin C fit into this equation? There are many studies that underscore the role of the ascorbates in tuberculosis, rabies, herpes, tetanus, poliomyelitis, and diphtheria.[2]

A Call To (Molecular) Arms

In the case of a national (political) crisis, there is a massive mobilization of men and machinery. They're readied for war. The situation in human survival is no different. When the organism is threatened by a foreign enemy, it responds with molecular mobilization. The military machinery is represented by many different chemical (also called humoral) substances. The ordnance consists of **immunoglobulins** (Ig), **prostaglandins,** and **interferon.** The manpower equivalent, the living cells, (the soldiers) are represented by the **phagocytes.**

How does vitamin C bolster our defense systems?

Prinz and his associates from the University of Witwatersrand Medical School gave one gram of ascorbic acid per day to 25 healthy male medical students over a period of 75 days.[3] These South African researchers emphasize several points. Vitamin C is vital for the antibodies IgA and IgM, and other humoral factors. On the other hand, the 20 subjects in the control-group not given the vitamin showed no change in the blood immunologic levels. Here's a clear example of the role of the ascorbates in the biologic ordnance system.

Another interesting report from South Africa was conducted by Anderson and his colleagues at the University of Pretoria.[4] They gave five healthy adults one gram of ascorbate each day of the first week, two grams daily the second week, and three grams on every day of the third week. These immunologists reported no change in the first week. But, with two or three grams of vitamin C, the important blood element called neutrophils swung quickly into action against bacterial toxins. What is particularly fascinating about this report, other than the importance of vitamin C and immunity, is that the dosage of ascorbic acid is much higher than generally reported in carefully supervised and controlled experiments of this type. Here's an excellent opportunity to witness the influence of AA on the health of the cellular soldiers.

Uncommon Outcomes of the Common Cold

Sir, in 1973 Olav J. Braendon, then at the UN Narcotics Laboratory in Geneva, published a ten-year study on Norwegian lumberjacks who did not have colds during periods spent in the mountains but were as susceptible as everyone else when they returned to the valleys. The preventive factor was found to lie in reducing substances emanating from the pinewood burnt in the primitive stoves in the cabins, and further research showed sodium ascorbate to be the most effective anti-toxicant . . . After discussion with a physiologist—I decided to put it to the test. At the beginning of what showed signs of becoming an especially nasty cold, I put some ascorbic acid powder up each nostril and sniffed in hard . . . Within 5 minutes the accumulated mucus turned liquid . . . I repeated the treatment . . . by lunchtime I felt fine . . .

Anne-Lisa Gotzche[5]

At the present time, the orthodox prevention and treatment of a common cold leaves much to be desired. The usual preventative recommendation is to avoid such victims. The therapy is nonspecific with bed rest, fluids, and the assurance that the syndrome is self-limiting. Hence, it is interesting to observe the mode of application of the case report just described.

The point was made in Chapter Two that vitamin C endured a long and dry season from about 1750 to the mid 1900s. Then, as you may remember, the story changed.

Doctor Linus Pauling says that he gradually became aware of the existence of an extraordinary contradiction between the opinions of different people about the value of vitamin C in preventing and ameliorating the common cold. Maxine Briggs[2] tabulates over 100 experiments, admittedly with varying results, of the relationship of the common cold to the ascorbates. Many people believe that vitamin C helps prevent colds; on the other hand, most physicians deny that C has much value. Accordingly, Doctor Pauling took the time and energy to examine the raw facts with the hope that there might be a valid reason for this obvious discrepancy. This, as we know now, was the basis for his book described earlier (Chapter Two).

There are others . . . Researchers from Australia

separated 95 pairs of identical twins into two groups.[6] One twin from each pair took a placebo every day. The other was administered 1000 mgs of vitamin C daily for a total of 100 days. The researchers from New South Wales found that in the vitamin C group there was a significantly shorter (19%) average duration of colds. At first blush, the results don't appear to be dramatic. Would they have been more pronounced with larger vitamin C dosage? Starting earlier? Providing ascorbic acid plus other agents (e.g. bioflavonoids)? In any case, within the limits of their observations, C made for kinder and gentler colds!

A more targeted series of observations. Enter Elliot Dick, Ph.D. Professor of Preventive Medicine and Director of the Respiratory Virus Research Laboratory at the University of Wisconsin-Madison.[7] He presented three trials at the fall 1990 session of the Interscience Conference on Antimicrobial Agents and Chemotherapy (ICAAC). These materials are to be published.

We'll dwell on these experiments in some detail because there is a great deal of confusion about the effectiveness of vitamin C supplementation in ameliorating or preventing common colds. This confusion is at least partly the result of the difficulty in managing a number of variables in previous trials including (a) a lack of adequate controls for the vitamin C status of the test subjects, (b) possible variability in the types of viruses infecting test and control subjects in open populations, and (c) adequately measuring a cold. These investigators developed an meticulous human volunteer model whereby laboratory-induced colds caused by a single **rhinovirus (RV)** serotype can be naturally transmitted to others at a predictable rate over a one-week period. The system allows nearly complete control over a small study population. In a series of three trials, they used this model to evaluate the effect of vitamin C supplementation upon naturally transmitted RV16 (a special species of colds).

In each of these three randomized double-blind trials, 16 healthy, nonsmoking adult male volunteers (we'll call them recipients), free of neutralizing antibody RV16, were given tablets containing either vitamin C (500 mg four times daily; n=8) or placebo (n=8). The recipients were dosed for 3.5 weeks and then housed for seven days with eight men (we'll call them donors) with deliberately laboratory-induced RV16 colds. During this week, the donors and recipients engaged in a variety of supervised interactions as well as sleeping, eating and studying in the same room. Vitamin C and placebo tablets were continued over the interaction period and the following two weeks. The 7-day donor-recipient interface period was chosen since, in prior experiments of this duration, nearly 100% of the recipients became infected.

Colds were detected by several methods. Hourly symptom diaries, in which a number of signs and symptoms were graded from 0 (absent) to 3 (severe) were kept by each recipient throughout the waking hours of the interaction period and the subsequent two weeks. A daily total symptom score (TSS) as well as a cumulative TSS for the entire study was then computed. In addition, during the contact period all volunteers were closely monitored 24 hours a day for clinical signs (coughs, sneezes and noseblows). Also, another sign, total mucus weight from tissues collected during the study, was included.

Finally, infection was detected by virus culture and

titration (to determine the amount of virus shed) of daily nasal washes taken during the period of interaction and through the two-week post-contact period, and by RV16 **seroconversion.**

Vitamin C levels in serum and purified mixed leukocytes were monitored weekly throughout each experiment, including three times during the interaction period. Furthermore, ascorbic acid levels were also measured in purified **granulocytes** and mononuclear cells.

The results are clear and best summarized by these researchers:

> Supplementation with vitamin C significantly decreased the severity of signs and symptoms of naturally-transmitted RV16 colds but did not prevent infection . . . The amelioration of RV16 illness was related to increased leukocyte vitamin C levels . . . These findings suggest that vitamin C supplementation may be useful for lessening disease severity as well as reducing virus transmission.

There is More Respiratory Disease than the Common Cold

Considerable attention has not only been paid to the common cold but also to other respiratory syndromes. As a matter of fact, we have already alluded to our studies of the health of members of the health profession.[8] Eight hundred and ninety dental practitioners and their spouses were studied on two occasions in terms of reported daily vitamin C consumption versus respiratory symptoms and signs (Figure 6.1). In the 410 (white column) with an average daily vitamin C intake of 332 mgs, there were no pulmonary complaints. In contrast, the 134 subjects with three or more respiratory findings (black column) showed the lowest mean ascorbic acid consumption of 275 mg. The intermediate groups, in terms of clinical symptomatology, are paralleled by intermediate scores of daily vitamin C consumption. From these data, it's convincingly clear that there's a significant relationship between daily vitamin C intake and nonspecific respiratory symptomatology.

Following the initial survey, health education lectures were provided to this group. This included discussions of the existing dietary patterns and possible changes that could and should be instituted. The group was re-examined the following year by the same tech-

Figure 6.1

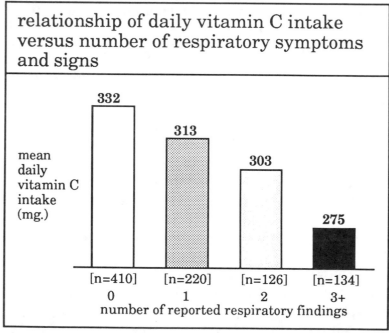

relationship of daily vitamin C intake versus number of respiratory symptoms and signs

mean daily vitamin C intake (mg.)

332	313	303	275
[n=410]	[n=220]	[n=126]	[n=134]
0	1	2	3+

number of reported respiratory findings

niques outlined previously. It is relevant to point out that well over three-fourths, actually 78.8% of the group, increased the daily vitamin C intake between the first and second visit. Additionally, the mean pulmonary score dropped about 25%. Clearly, not everybody increased their C intake the same. A comparison of the respiratory findings in those who stepped up their ascorbic acid to 400+ versus those who didn't showed a difference in respiratory improvement of about 50%.

The evidence suggests that vitamin C is not only helpful for the common cold but the overall pulmonary picture.

The New Bug on the Block

There are thousands and thousands of different microbes. With regard to humans, most are harmless; some are actually helpful; others even necessary. The ones we hear the most about include a relatively small group that play havoc. Within this last group, there's a smaller set known to be sexually-transmitted. We have all heard of syphilis, gonorrhea and others.

But there's a new bug on the block. Only in the very last few years have we learned of the acronym AIDS (Acquired Immune Deficiency Syndrome) presumably due to HIV (Human Immunodeficiency Virus). It first became popularly recognized among homosexuals. However, it is now conceded that the problem can be transmitted by infected needles, blood transfusions, and with heterosexual behavior.

Its uniqueness doesn't end here. There is great interest as evidenced by approximately six thousand scientific published articles during the last year. The former U. S. Surgeon General, Doctor Everett Koop, has warned that about one hundred million people worldwide could die from AIDS by the year 2000 if a solution isn't found. It is obviously increasingly common and clearly deadly. At the present time, there are no preventative vaccines and the current therapies are few and expensive. Their effectiveness is even questioned.

There is an increasing body of fact suggesting significant relationships between AIDS and a number of vitamins and minerals. This information has been summarized in a review entitled *Preventive Health Care for Adults with HIV Infection.*[9] Interestingly, the major thrust has been vitamin A, B complex, zinc, selenium and copper. As far as we can determine, there is very little information about the ascorbates.

Notwithstanding, we learned in Chapter Five that vitamin C acts as an electron donor. It was also discovered at that time that it's a potent antioxidant and serves a scavenger role. This point has been applied to the AIDS issue in an unpublished paper.[10]

> The overlooked idea is that massive doses of ascorbate can actually be the source of high-energy electrons used in the process of free radical scavenging and not just an electron carrier used repeatedly in an electron-transport-chain resulting in free radical scavenging.

As far as we can determine, Robert F. Cathcart, III, M.D. has probably the greatest clinical experience with the use of the ascorbates with AIDS. He has expressed himself clearly on this point.[11-12]

My previous experience with the utilization of ascorbic acid in the treatment of viral diseases led me to hypothesize that ascorbate would be of value in the treatment of AIDS. Preliminary clinical evidence is that massive doses of ascorbate (50-200 grams per 24 hours) can markedly reduce the tendency for secondary infections . . . The AIDS patient who has already suffered a marked suppression of (immunity), presents a clinical problem of management similar to a bubble baby . . . The patient who takes (massive) doses of ascorbic acid, may remain clinically well . . . There have been suggestive anecdotal cases which indicate that in the prodromal period, before the destruction of (immunity) there might be avoidance of the development of the AIDS syndrome by this program.

We will not deal with the subject in great detail in this book principally because there are no sharply defined and carefully supervised controlled experiments. In the interest of accuracy and completeness, we must note that there are isolated reports to encourage the use of the ascorbates. As representative of the work being done, we mention interesting in-vitro studies from the Linus Pauling Institute of Science and Medicine.[13-14] This group notes the suppression of virus production in HIV infected cells grown in the presence of nontoxic concentrations of ascorbate. Such observations are consistent with the antiviral activity of vitamin C against a broad spectrum of viruses both in humans and in the test tube.

Summary and Conclusions

It is time to lay to rest the notion that germs jump into people and cause diseases. The evidence is adequate that microbes challenge the internal milieu. The end-result depends upon the organism's ability to resist by means of its army of defense systems. They come under different names and serve diverse purposes. What is common is that they protect us against the relentless noxious microbial invasion.

The data suggest that, if and when enough work has been done, vitamin C will contribute to an effective defense against infectious states.

So, *Vitamin C . . . who needs it?* W. J. McCormick from Canada recognized and reported its benefits way back in 1952 in his statement:[15]

When 500 to 1000 mg doses are given intravenously or intramuscularly every hour or two, the effects compare favorably with those resulting from antibiotics that are routinely prescribed . . . Spectacular results have been achieved in pneumonia, tuberculosis, scarlet fever, pelvic infections and septicemia.

Obviously, infections continue to be critical. However, with the increasing life expectancy, there has been a shift in disease patterns. As more and more people tend to live longer, the chronic degenerative disorders are gaining in importance. Hence, it seems wise to now turn our attention to the ascorbates in our common killing and crippling syndromes. This will be the emphasis in the next chapter.

7

COMMON KILLERS
AND CRIPPLERS

What do cardiovascular (heart and blood vessel) disease and cancer have in common?

More than you may think!

For one, these two groups constitute some of our current major killing and crippling fears. Secondly, there is considerable dissatisfaction by the public as well as the professions with their present solutions.

- In one day, 4,100 Americans suffer a heart attack and 1,500 die.

- Of every 100 American deaths, 35 are due to heart disease.

- There are 500 coronary bypass operations performed each day. This makes it a $3.5 billion a year business.

• It is, in fact, the most common major surgical procedure in this country.

Now to carcinomatosis . . .

• There are over six million living Americans who have a history of malignancies.

• It kills more children age 3 to 14 than any other disease.

• According to the American Cancer Society (ACS), about 83 million persons now alive in this country will contract cancer — "about one in three."[1]

• The ACS predicted that in 1992, 1,130,000 new cases would be diagnosed in the U.S.

• In Cancer Facts and Figures—1992, "the five year survival rate is only 13% in all patients, regardless of stage at diagnosis." Match this against the fact that the federal government has spent an estimated $22 billion on the war against cancer in the past 20 years.

From these figures, it is fairly obvious that we need a hard and fresh look for more preventive and therapeutic answers.

The possible explanations for both of these sets of diseases are largely epidemiologic. (Meaning convincing relationships and not necessarily cause-and-effect.)

But, what is particularly exciting is that diet is increasingly a lead player in the story. Regrettably, there are relatively few sophisticated double-blind studies to nail down causation. Some of the reasons are obvious. People with such problems are usually very sick and, therefore, frequently do not lend themselves to fancy experimentation and dummy pills. There is also the obvious morality issue.

Finally, when one examines the mechanisms by which vitamin C operates, it looks like the processes involved in cancer and cardiovascular disease are the same or similar. These two devastating sets of problems have in common disturbances in lipid metabolism. Heavily implicated, as has already been mentioned (Chapter Five), is the free radical phenomenon.

The New Word in the Old Word Game!

We have all been amused with the stimulus/response pastime. Say black and the answer is generally white, hot—cold and so on. Pose the word heart disease and out pops cholesterol. The point of the story is that the public has now been educated to the strong relationship between the lipids and cardiovascular disease (CVD). It has gotten so simplified that all one need do is to cut out cholesterol to cut out heart disease. We learn from Matthias Rath (mentioned earlier in Chapter Two) that one of the most significant consequences of hypoascorbemia is blood vessel collapse. Incidentally it is noteworthy that premature CVD is essentially unknown in all animal species that produce their own high amounts of C. Humans, for protection, have strengthened the blood vessels with certain fats.

And now it seems that maybe the single most important lipid buzzword is lipoprotein a (Lp-a).[2-4] But the critical item is that the higher the C, the lower the Lp-a! We will mention more regarding its connection to cardiovascular disease, cancer, and diabetes in later sections.

The Silent Beginning

We have all heard of the woman who (seemingly) suddenly notes a lump in her breast. Well-known is the man who (seemingly) suddenly breaks out in a sweat and excruciating chest pain. What is not so obvious is that these seemingly sudden experiences are anything but sudden. They are slow and insidious. One of the reflections of this long and silent period is a reduction in energy reserve. In other words, the patient notes with time fatigability variously described as exhaustion, tiredness or lassitude.

There is abundant hindsight evidence from recovered heart attack victims. About three out of four persons will tell you that inordinate fatigue was the single most dominant warning of their impending problem. And one of the mirrors of that energy problem can be measured by heart rate. This point is described in the following experiment.

A group of Dutch investigators have been studying the effect of marginal vitamin C deficiency states on performance. In one of their experiments,[5] these scientists from the Departments of Human Nutrition and Clinical Biochemistry performed a double-blind study on the effects of vitamin C restriction on physical performance in 12 deemed-to-be healthy men. During seven weeks of low vitamin C intake, six subjects were on a daily diet of regular food products, providing 20% of the Dutch Recommended Dietary Allowances for vitamin C (the Dutch daily RDA is 50 mg). After three weeks of low vitamin intake an additional dose of 15 mg/day was provided, resulting in a total intake of 25 mg/day (50% of the Dutch RDA). Six control subjects consumed the same diet supplemented with twice the RDA for all vitamins. As one might expect, in the restricted group, blood vitamin C levels decreased significantly.

Then why the fuss? Under these conditions, the pulse rate increased. How much? Only about eight beats per minute. Hardly worth mentioning? But, this means eight times 60 equals 480 beats more per hour . . . 11,520 extra per day . . . over 4,000,000 per year . . . so, a little less vitamin C might mean 40,000,000 additional for the next decade. In other words, it looks like a marginal ascorbic acid deficit may invite a tremendous extra heart workload!

So, it may well be that the heart disease of today began way back then with a minimal hypoascorbemia!

Is There a Doctor in the Supermarket?

There are other seemingly silent beginnings.

Millions of considered-to-be healthy individuals are so concerned about their blood pressure that they want it checked at the most bizarre times and in the strangest places. This means in the supermarket . . . the drug store . . . and would-you-believe even at the launderette?

A great deal has been written and much blame has been placed for high blood pressure. What about the ascorbates? Several medical surveys of presumably healthy people have reported an inverse relationship between vitamin C status and resting blood pressure. It seems that the greater the vitamin C intake, the lower the blood pressure. But there are very few reports on what happens under carefully-controlled causation-oriented conditions.

In order to clarify this issue, a group from the Alcorn State University in Mississippi in a joint effort with the Beltsville Human Nutrition Research Center carried out the following experiment.[6] A tablet of 1000 mg ascorbic acid or a placebo was supplied daily to 20 adults for two six-week periods in a randomized, crossover design. The subjects consumed self-selected diets and were in presumably good vitamin C status. Twelve were classified as borderline hypertensive. Under these conditions, AA supplementation reduced systolic blood pressure but did not affect the diastolic state. In their own words, "It appears that vitamin C supplementation may have therapeutic value in human hypertensive disease."

Could the systolic pressure change be even greater with more vitamin C? Might there not also be a diastolic reduction? These and other burning questions are still to be answered.

The Sticky Story Revisited

We summarized earlier the importance of platelet function to health and sickness in general and clotting in particular (Chapter Five). Obviously, under homeostatic conditions, the quality and quantity of platelets should be such as to contribute to coagulation when indicated and to protect against such clotting when warranted. Bordia (we heard about him earlier in Chapter Five), in India, provides us with two excellent not-too-well-known experiments.[7] One is acute; the other of a chronic nature.

Forty patients with recent **myocardial infarction** were divided into two subsets. One received two grams of vitamin C daily for 20 days and the other was administered a placebo. Ascorbic acid blood samples were collected. Ascorbate administration increased fibrinolytic activity (blood thinning) by 63% while serum ascorbic acid rose 94%.

The second, the chronic, experiment embraces 40 patients with a past history of myocardial infarctions. This set was divided into three groups. The first subgroup served as controls while Groups II and III were given respectively, a total of one and two grams of vitamin C daily. Blood samples were collected initially, and then every two months during the six-month period of ascorbic acid administration and finally 60 days after cessation of supplementation. The ascorbates, 500 mg twice daily (Group II), increased serum AA by about 22%. However, no alterations were observed in fibrinolytic activity. Thus, under these conditions, no changes in blood clotting occurred. However, when the dose of C was doubled, (Group III), three important events followed. First, serum ascorbic acid rose by about 96%. Secondly, fibrinolysis increased 45%. Lastly, other measures of blood thinning (platelet adhesive index) confirmed these findings. In other words, utilizing this (generally conceded-to-be) relatively large vitamin C supplement, the blood picture favorably improved for heart patients.

What does all this mean?

First, these simple studies confirm what was described earlier (Chapter Five). In other words, it emphasizes the point that vitamin C plays an important role in platelet health. Secondly, it underlines the fact that this mechanism operates very quickly with benefits in a matter of days. Next, it makes the point that dosage does indeed play a significant role. With amounts approximating twelve times the RDA (one gram per day), the findings are negative. Doubling the doses of C (about 25 times the RDA) to two grams convincingly shows favorable blood-thinning benefits. Fourth, from these experiments, one must wonder how much more success could be derived by even greater and longer AA supplementation. Clearly, this observation must await further study.

On the other hand, there is the bigger picture. As a matter of record, each year the *Journal of the American Medical Association* (JAMA) devotes one of its issues to a summary of medical progress (or lack thereof) during that year. Such a review of cardiovascular disease has been recently published.[8] The principal thrust this year has been the search for better preventative and therapeutic solutions to the clotting phenomenon. In their own words:

> . . . There is still no consensus as to the most appropriate thrombolytic agent . . .

(In other words, the search is still on for better blood thinning factors.) Sadly, the thrombolytic utility of the ascorbates hasn't been examined seriously in spite of the evidence presented earlier in this chapter. Isn't vitamin C a reasonable alternative to the baby aspirin?

The Cancer Connection

Throughout the literature, and for many years past, there have been interesting epidemiologic (correlative) observations to suggest an exciting connection between diet in general and vitamin C in particular in carcinomatosis. Gladys Block of the National Cancer Institute presented a monumental piece of work at recent conferences in London and Washington, D. C. and subsequently published her findings.[9] Her report tabulated and summarized all of the available epidemiologic surveys of the role of vitamin C in carcinomatosis. We will delay detailed comment for a more appropriate time (Chapter Thirteen).

For the moment, it is important to mention that cancer tissue liberates an enzyme called hyaluronidase which dissolves, hyaluronic acid and thus invites the spread of tumors. It was based on this observation that Linus Pauling and his colleagues reached the conclusion that vitamin C should be of value in controlling cancer. The hypothesis is predicated on the fact that more collagen fibrils would be formed providing a more effective wall against the spread of the tumor.

Because of these observations, they carried out a series of experiments of vitamin C in patients with advanced cancer.[10-12]

Perhaps the most significant piece of work centers on one hundred terminal cancer patients given supplemental ascorbate matched against a control group. In other words, if there was a 46-year old white woman with a particular type of tumor in the supplemented group, she was compared against ten such females of the same age with the same cancer problem. It should be underlined that both the control and experimental groups were treated by the same clinicians in the same hospital and had been managed identically except for the additional ascorbates. All examinations were done by an independent practitioner so as to eliminate bias. The results, to say the least, were surprising. For example, the one hundred ascorbate-treated patients lived on the average about three hundred days longer than their matched controls. Those given vitamin C survived about one year longer! (Incidentally, this portion of the study was repeated with essentially the same results.) In the words of these investigators:

> We considered this to be a remarkable achievement, bearing in mind that if the mortality of cancer could be decreased by five percent, the lives of 20,000 American cancer patients would be saved each year.

The condition of the patients improved to such an extent that their lives during their remaining months or years were more comfortable, contented, useful, productive and satisfying. This was borne out in many ways including the fact that there was much less need for pain-killing medication.

As one might expect, there aren't too many such experiments. But, it is noteworthy that much of the epidemiologic background supports the studies just described (Chapter Thirteen).

Still Another Vitamin C Eye-Opener

What has not been mentioned thus far is that these killing and crippling diseases frequently eventuate in surgery. So, this invites an additional crisis, namely the hypoascorbemia state under such stress related conditions.

William W. Coon from the Department of Surgery at

the University of Michigan at Ann Arbor studied the whole blood and buffy coat ascorbic acid levels of 130 patients undergoing major abdominal surgery.[13] He confirmed the characteristic drop in the blood levels during the first several postoperative days. Accordingly, this Michigan investigator provided different groups of patients with different amounts of vitamin C. One subset was given nothing, another 75, 100, 150, 200, or even 300 mg of the ascorbates daily by subcutaneous (under the skin) injection. Utilizing 0.4 mg% as an acceptable blood level (and this, as we know, can be challenged), he concluded that 200 mg of ascorbic acid must be given daily parenterally (injection) to compensate for the stress conditions. We should recall our earlier discussion (Chapter Four) indicating that a more desirable blood concentration would be 1.0 mg%.

On the basis of his findings, it is clear that most patients undergoing surgery require more vitamin C than generally administered. What is not certain is how much more the average person under these conditions needs. Obviously, the final word hasn't yet been written. It would seem that it's probably more likely in gram concentrations.

In any case, we find here a double jeopardy situation. Patients with serious diseases may need more of the ascorbates. Additionally, the solution to their problem (i.e. surgery) may set an added vitamin C load.

Summary and Conclusions

This chapter, more than any thus far and even to come, is brimming with death and drama and fraught with great difficulty and delicacy.

The deadliness is obvious. The drama stems from the exciting possibility that a simple nutrient can favorably effect extraordinary changes in the prevention and treatment of cardiovascular disease and carcinomatosis.

However, there is a price to pay. The fact that the critical situation can be terminal and devastating makes it technically difficult and sometimes morally unconscionable to carry out the most desired research procedures including the famous double-blind crossover studies. While such opportunities are limited, the data here plus the added information (Chapter Thirteen) collectively suggest that there are powerful relationships between the ascorbates and these deadly disorders.

All of this should be weighed against recent figures by the Pharmaceutical Manufacturers Association.[14] They give us the numbers for the current research efforts for drug products. Cardiovascular agents received the greatest single research monies in 1989 and to the tune of 23%. Neoplasms ranked second with 15.2%. Vitamins were only accorded 0.2%!

While the unhappy news is that there is a paucity of studies, there's the flipside, the good news. It's comforting to know that these presumed to be seemingly separate and distinct sets of syndromes (cardiovascular pathosis and cancer) can both be to some degree prevented and treatmentwise aided by this single nutrient.

Finally, the very solutions to our most killing and crippling diseases frequently require surgery. We now know that the ascorbates may overcome these stress-related circumstances.

Hence, *Vitamin C . . . who needs it?* As for the

killers and cripplers, everybody does for two reasons. First, the evidence presented in this chapter. Second, the alternatives are so poor. And so, what's there to lose? Third, in a study of 15,871 persons who reported being treated for high blood cholesterol, 79% indicated that a low-fat or low-cholesterol diet had been recommended, 19% confirmed that lipid-lowering medication had been prescribed, and 20% reported that they had been referred to a dietitian or other health professional for dietary counseling. Here in 1993, we have reasonable confirmation of the continuing inattention to the ascorbates.[15]

There are other very disabling problems. One of cardinal interest and apparently increasingly so is the subject of diabetes mellitus. This will be our focus in the next chapter.

3

DIABETES AND SCURVY: ARE THEY COUSINS?

There is no monopoly on dreadful and devastating disorders (Chapter Seven). A good example is diabetes mellitus. It is of concern for two reasons. First, the diabetic state, in its own right, can play metabolic havoc. Second, diabetes mellitus is a risk factor for those killing and crippling fears described earlier. It's well-known that the diabetic state often precedes many different cardiovascular and cancer syndromes.

Just about all of the experts view diabetes mellitus as a common malady. The old, conservative, very traditional, but still cited number is that one in one hundred Americans are known victims; another one percent is not aware they suffer with this metabolic disease.[1] The orthodox view is that two percent of the population is diabetic. However, there are other, widely differing estimates. Professor T.S. Danowski,[2] a celebrated endocrinologist at the University of Pittsburgh, made the following point:

> Approximately, one out of four people, in the course of a lifetime, develops diabetes or episodes of hyperglycemia that are indistinguishable from diabetes. This means 25% of the population, not 2%, which has been the general impression. The higher figure comes from consecutive studies of individuals from birth to death, rather than the prevalence rate in a given community at a given time.

Whatever the true number, lots of people are afflicted with this metabolic malady. Moreover, with more people living longer, the figure in the elderly seems to be rising rapidly.

Finally, one need not look too far to learn that the present preventative and therapeutic approach to the diabetic state leaves much to be desired.

• Between 1965 and 1973, the prevalence of diabetes increased more than 50% in the U.S.A.

• During the 12-month period from March 1989 to March 1990, an estimated 13.2 million visits were made to office-based physicians in the United States, at which the principal, or first-listed diagnosis was diabetes mellitus. An additional 8.7 million visits included diabetes mellitus as the second or third listed diagnosis.[3]

• Anyone born today who lives an average life span of 70 years has greater than a one in five chance of developing this killer disease!

• After 20 years of diabetes, 45% of diabetics have peripheral vascular disease.

• The lowest cost estimates attributable directly to diabetes are $13.5 billion annually, about 3.6% of the so-called total health expenses in the U.S.

These data all suggest that it might be time to look to a new philosophy and a hard and fresh scrutiny of diabetes mellitus.

Where to begin?

The Case of the Diabetic Pig

We learned way back there (Chapter Two) that only a very few animals are incapable of manufacturing their own vitamin C. As a matter of fact, it's this that makes the guinea pig and man cousins. So, it should be no surprise that a long time ago (1936) Sigal[4] carried out one of those exciting experiments by treating the guinea pig as if it were a human organism. He simply took a group of healthy pigs and denied them vitamin C while studying the glucose tolerance pattern. Figure 8.1 shows that after a mere ten days, the glucose tolerance curve began to approach that of a diabetic. In other words, at each temporal point the blood sugar is higher. With further ascorbate restriction, the pattern systematically worsened.

Here is a clear and simple demonstration of the connection between vitamin C and the diabetic process.

Figure 8.1

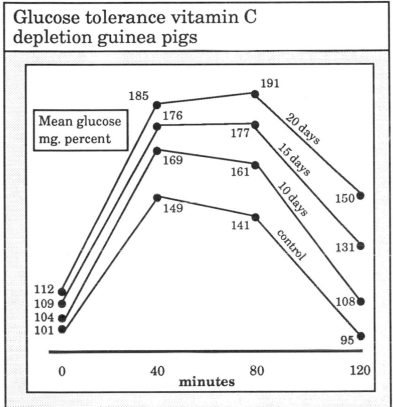

Glucose tolerance vitamin C
depletion guinea pigs

Mean glucose
mg. percent

191
185
176
177
20 days
15 days
169
161
10 days
150
149
141
control
131
112
109
104
101
108
95

0   40   80   120
minutes

A Simple and Successful
Piece of the Puzzle

We are all aware of the wonders of the cardiovascular system. It has been pictured as a tree with many branches. These can be divided into two parts. On the one hand, there's the heart and the major blood vessels (arteries, arterioles, venules and veins). Their prime purpose is to serve as a freeway (transport) system. They guarantee to deliver the blood to all parts of the body. But, the critical areas are the off-freeway-ramps (the capillaries). It's at these points that the much-needed nutrients and oxygen are delivered to the tissues and the unnecessary metabolites removed.

During fetal development, the brain grows in such a way that one of its terminations is the eyeballs. It is with good reason that the doctor looks into the eye with a special lighted instrument. Here's where the physician can actually examine directly the blood vessels of the eye which, in effect, are the small vessels of the brain.

We have already learned (Chapter Two) that there are simple and reasonable informative tests to measure capillary fragility and permeability. Finally, what's important to emphasize is that these simple measurements in the skin of small blood vessel health are equally reflective of the capillary state in the eye.

British researchers, B. D. Cox and W. J. H. Butterfield studied the small blood vessels of the skin and retina (the back side of the eye) of 24 normal subjects and 12 diabetics.[5] These investigators made the point that the average diabetic gets about half the average amount of vitamin C (meaning 1/4 that of the typical nondiabetic). They report the not-too-well-known observation that diabetics show much more fragile capillaries that rupture easily. This is one of the reasons why diabetics have so much eye trouble.

For treatment, the diabetics were assigned to two groups in a crossover study. Category One was given a placebo for one month, then vitamin C (one gram per day) for two months. Group Two was provided vitamin C supplementation (one gram/day) for two months then placebo for one month. Every 30 days, skin capillary fragility was assessed, blood vitamin C estimated, and the fundi (eye blood vessels) examined. The results suggest that the capillaries in diabetics are more fragile than nondiabetics. What is significant here is that the experiment revealed very clearly that the capillary strength of all diabetics improved during the vitamin C treatment. When the ascorbates were withdrawn in Group Two, the capillary strength deteriorated toward the end of the month. It should also come as no surprise that the retinal blood picture pretty much followed the cutaneous story.

This exciting and simple experiment makes a number of very critical points. It is obvious that diabetics, as a group, consume less vitamin C. Hence, one must wonder whether, in fact, there would be fewer diabetic patients if the general intake of ascorbic acid were greater. (And remember, as discussed in Chapter Four, Mr. and Mrs. Average American consume about half the vitamin C they should.) There's the interesting dimension of measurement and by a relatively simple technique, namely capillary strength. But, sadly as we'll see later in this chapter, ascorbate supplementation is not even a part of diabetic orthodoxy.

It is generally known that the diabetic is prone to many complications, the common denominator being blood vessel health. The literature is replete with evidences of the ravages of diabetic gangrene. It occurs 25 times more readily in diabetics than in nondiabetics. Also, the horrors of diabetic **nephropathy** are well-established.

One must wonder what might happen to all these complications if the daily vitamin C supplementation was increased several fold. Obviously, the answer will have to await additional experimentation.

Other Cousinly Connections?

One of the many myths in modern medicine centers on the notion that specific biochemical states represent specific clinical syndromes. By act, if not by word, there's the crazy idea that a high blood cholesterol specifically means heart disease. There is lots of literature to suggest that an elevated uric acid is the biochemical label for gout. And most appropriately here, we make our diabetic diagnoses from the blood sugar. Not true. Most biochemical parameters characterize many different clinical states.

Emil Ginter of the Institute of Human Nutrition in Bratislava and his colleagues make the well-established point that a significantly lower vitamin C concentration has been found in the blood and particularly the leukocytes of hypercholesterolemic (high cholesterol) diabetic patients when compared to that of healthy blood donors.[6] This Czech doctor reported the vitamin C leukocyte levels were two and one half times greater in non-diabetics. In the light of these observations, he administered ascorbic acid in a dose of 500 mg/day for 12 months to maturity-onset diabetics. These were fairly controlled subjects on a standard diabetic diet not requiring insulin or any other heroic drugs. The results are clear as judged by a striking decline of hypercholesterolemia and a moderate reduction of triglycerides. The serum lipid level in a matched control group given placebo remained unaltered.

Here we have a very simple demonstration of the cholesterol-lowering effect of the ascorbates confirming once again the versatility of vitamin C (Chapter Five).

The "For-Your-Age" Myth

We will be devoting an entire section to the aging process and especially the role of the ascorbates in the geriatric state. For the moment, our concern here is with aging in the light of carbohydrate metabolism and the diabetic phenomenon.

Notwithstanding the palaver, in the final analysis whether a patient is deemed a diabetic or not is derived from the testing of blood sugar. Different experts utilize different methods for measuring blood glucose. Without becoming involved in all the particulars, the most sophisticated approach to the assessment of carbohydrate metabolism is one of the several types of glucose tolerance tests. All of them have in common that the metabolic state is first challenged by a glucose load (meaning the injection or ingestion of a known amount of a simple carbohydrate). This then is followed by the measurement of blood glucose at several subsequent temporal points.

There is great confusion as to where one draws the line between the diabetic and the nondiabetic. Part of the chaos stems from the use of different glucose challenges. Some doctors provide the patient with 50 or 100 grams or different amounts based on body weight. Such different challenges obviously modify the resultant blood glucose picture. But the single biggest problem stems from an assumption that, as one gets older, the acceptable blood glucose is higher.

No question, it is a fact that just about every blood glucose survey shows that, with advancing age, the blood glucose rises. We've confirmed this point in the Birmingham (Alabama) 1964 Diabetes Detection Drive by means of a study of 8940 participants ranging in age from 9 to 91 years.[7] Table 8.1 shows convincingly

Table 8.1
Age and capillary blood sugar

age groups	sample size	capillary blood sugar (mg.%)
0-19	919	85
20-39	1750	85
40-59	3680	89
60-79	2473	92
80-99	84	95

that the lowest blood glucose (85 mg%) parallels the youngest group; the highest blood sugar in the oldest (95 mg%).

Hence, within this ten-decade age range, the blood sugar rises on the average about 10 mg%. It looks as though one can expect, on an average basis, an insidious one milligram percent increment in blood glucose per decade. Put in real terms, some people rise more, others less.

We have also examined the relationship of age and carbohydrate metabolism by means of the Cortisone Glucose Tolerance Test in 169 apparently healthy individuals.[8] The group was arbitrarily divided into two subsets based upon age. There were 89 subjects under 36 years of age; 80 above. Table 8.2 summarizes the blood glucose levels in these two groups at all temporal points. For example, under fasting conditions, the younger set showed a blood glucose of 79 mg%; the older 85 mg%. Hence, even under fasting conditions here is already a significant difference of 6 mg%. You will find that this same pattern prevails throughout, namely, that older individuals tend to have higher, probably poorer, blood sugar concentrations.

Table 8.2

The relationship of age and the cortisone glucose tolerance pattern in relatively young (under 36 yrs.) and old (36+ yrs.) subjects		
cortisone glucose tolerance test	younger (n=89) mean	older (n=80) mean
fasting	79	85
30 minute	132	141
1 hour	127	150
2 hours	96	115
3 hours	75	89

As we have just noted, the fact of the matter is that there is indeed a positive correlation between age and blood glucose. It's this fact that has led to the conclusion that this phenomenon is "normal." It is certainly the case if one defines "normality" as "average." However, is "normality" also "optimal?"

In other words, we now know that blood glucose seems to rise with age in ordinary subjects. The new and different question is "Does blood glucose rise with age in 'healthy' persons?"

To resolve this question, we returned to the 169 normal, generally thought-to-be-healthy, individuals who were subjected to one type of procedure (the then popular Cortisone-Glucose-Tolerance Test).[8] These subjects were divided into near-equal subsets based upon their plasma AA state. There were 103 people with plasma levels less than 0.6 mg%. We will arbitrarily refer to this group as in relatively poorer ascorbate condition. This is based on our earlier observations (Chapter Four). The remaining 66 were characterized by a blood plasma of 0.6+ mg%. These will be hereafter referred to as the better ascorbate group.

Table 8.3 summarizes the blood glucose levels based upon poorer vitamin C state in younger versus older

Table 8.3

The relationship of age and the cortisone glucose tolerance pattern in subjects with relatively poorer (<0.6 mg.%) ascorbate state

cortisone glucose tolerance test	age <36 years	age <36+ years
fasting	77	88
30 minute	134	148
1 hour	129	158
2 hours	97	121
3 hours	74	92

subjects. For example, under fasting conditions the blood glucose was 77 in the younger and 88 in the older. Hence, the findings earlier described for the entire group are confirmed here (a difference of 11 mg%). The same pattern prevails throughout. In other words, the blood glucose does indeed rise with age in those with the suboptimal vitamin C conditions.

If this is true then an analysis of blood glucose shouldn't advance with time in those endowed with a satisfactory ascorbate state. To check this hypothesis, Table 8.4 is provided.

Table 8.4

The relationship of age and the cortisone glucose tolerance pattern in subjects with relatively good (>0.6 mg.%) ascorbate state		
cortisone glucose tolerance test	age <36 years	age <36+ years
fasting	82	80
30 minute	129	130
1 hour	123	139
2 hours	94	107
3 hours	77	84

Under fasting conditions, the blood glucose is 82 and 80 mg% in the younger and older groups respectively. This pattern seems to prevail throughout. Hence, we have the additional confirmation that blood glucose doesn't ordinarily rise significantly with age in relatively healthier subjects.

To the extent that one can draw conclusions, it is indeed a myth to believe that as one gets older the diabetic potential rises. The fact of the matter is that as one gets older the diabetic potential increases in subjects under suboptimal ascorbate conditions. Here's a bit more evidence of the cousinly connection!

Summary and Conclusions

Implied, if not stated, is that there are two major groups of killing and crippling disorders. Now we learn that, in fact, there are more. Diabetes mellitus, in its own right, plays great havoc. Also, it sets the stage for the ravages of cardiovascular diseases and carcinomatosis.

The evidence presented here, while admittedly limited, suggests that manifestations of the diabetic state can be significantly altered with changes in the ascorbates. We had the opportunity to confirm this with regard to capillary (both skin and eye) strength. We have also noted significant biochemical (lipid) alterations.

Finally, there is evidence that vitamin C may also be useful in a preventive sense as judged by the shape of the glucose tolerance pattern.

So, what do the experts tell us about a vitamin C connection in the control of sugar metabolism?

We turned to five of the leading textbooks dealing with diabetes mellitus published during the last five years.[9-13] Would you believe? There was not one word indicating any connection—or a lack of correlation—between ascorbic acid and carbohydrate metabolism!

This is even more incomprehensible when one realizes that reviews of the literature as far back as 1940[14] showed that blood sugar can be predictably reduced with intravenous ascorbate. But perhaps the following anecdote will cinch the story.

Dice and Daniel of Stanford University comment on their own experiences.[15] Doctor Dice, who had been diagnosed as diabetic at age fifteen, served as his own guinea pig in this experiment. Unresponsive to then-popular pills for lowering blood sugar, he was taking insulin by injection. To test the C connection, he took progressively increasing amounts of ascorbic acid each hour from 7 A.M. to 1 A.M. When hypoglycemia (lowered blood sugar) occurred, he cut the daily amount of insulin. When glycosuria (sugar in the urine) developed, he added more vitamin C. In this small study, it was shown "that ascorbic acid exhibits marked glycemic activity."

So, *Vitamin C . . . who needs it?* According to conventional thinking . . . apparently nobody. However, in light of the limited studies cited here and backed up by much in the literature, every diabetic or potential candidate would be well-served by adding vitamin C to their therapeutic and preventative armamentarium.

9

A MOUTHFUL
OF EVIDENCE

Who among us hasn't heard (possibly even to the point of nausea) the time-honored adage, "Those who cannot remember the past are condemned to repeat it?" The saga of scurvy in stomatology is a superlative case.

You will recall the earlier stories concerning sea voyages. The point was made even back then of a trinity of symptomatology, namely inordinate weakness, the hemorragic diathesis, and spongy (and clearly bleeding) gums. So, we've long known of the connection between vitamin C state and the oral tissues.

Second, this chapter is also unique because it deals with the number one twentieth-century chronic problem in western culture. No question . . . 95% of the public suffers with dental caries and/or periodontal disease.

There is also another, and very exciting, uniqueness

to stomatology. Mention was made (Chapter Five) that disease is the result of the interplay of a constellation of environmental challenges as it relates to the internal milieu. The oral cavity is one of the few areas where experiments can be performed delineating the relative importance of the environment and host state. For example, it's possible to clean and polish only half the teeth (e.g. the right or left side). This then allows a comparison of the effect of modifying the local environment versus letting it remain unchanged. On the other hand, you can give a group of subjects vitamin C versus a placebo. (We tried but failed to give half a person ascorbate!) By these experimental designs, one can derive the relative contributions of these four different ecologic possibilities. There is also the converse. Banding half the teeth makes it possible to compare the added irritation (of bands versus no bands) in the light of vitamin C and placebo supplementation. Such experiments have been described in the literature with various nutrients including ascorbic acid. We'll return to these studies later in this chapter.

The Current Official Dental Opinion

Russell in 1963 summarized the results of the studies conducted under the auspices of the Interdepartmental Committee for Nutrition in National Defense (ICNND). They recorded the dietary and oral health status of selected samples.[1] The evaluation of nutritional deficiencies was based on clinical examinations and on biochemical tests of blood and urine in a small subsample. Serum levels of ascorbic acid were used in the ICNND studies to assess deficiency levels. You will recall that the ICNND played a big role in the original standards for blood AA concentrations (Chapter Four). Russell concluded from these well-publicized epidemiologic data that age and oral hygiene (we'll examine carefully this term later) contributed most to the variance in Periodontal Index (PI) scores. Also, he further concluded no correlation between ascorbic acid deficiency and increased PI scores (the then most popular measure of periodontal health). In another study, the Ten State Nutrition Survey, only a "weak" correlation was reported between hypoascorbemia and the presence of gum disease.[2]

These observations in the 60s dominated and continue to color the thinking of dentistry. It even serves today as a basis for the relative unimportance of the ascorbates in oral health and sickness.

On the other hand, there have been, and still are, many clinicians who feel from their limited but presumably cause-and-effect observations that vitamin C seems to play a role in oral health. For these reasons plus the fact that a large governmental study had been completed, it became possible to reexamine the epidemiologic data.

This project[3] investigated the association (again in an epidemiologic way) between the reported levels of dietary ascorbic acid intake and the presence of periodontal disease. A representative segment of the U.S. population provided by the first National Health and Nutrition Examination Survey (NHANES I), from 1971 to 1974 was reviewed. The NHANES I survey was a comprehensive accounting of health and nutrition in more than 20,000 individuals, aged 1 to 74, in the continental United States. Data were collected from 8,609 dentulous (with teeth) persons, aged 25 to 74 years, who received a dental examination during NHANES I and with whom a 24-hour dietary recall interview was conducted. The purpose of this analysis was to investigate the possible correlation between periodontal disease and reported dietary intake of vitamin C. A corollary aim was to determine whether a more-than-recommended daily intake of ascorbic acid was associated with better periodontal health.

Periodontal disease status (PI) and oral hygiene state (Simplified Oral Hygiene Index, OHI-S), in addition to other oral and dental health assessments, were collected by ten trained dentists at 65 locations during the four years of the NHANES I survey.

Ascorbic acid intake was calculated from the foods putatively consumed by each individual during the preceding 24 hours. To insure the greatest possible accuracy, the interviews were conducted by persons trained in gathering dietary data. Parenthetic mention should be made that, in this report, the term "dietary ascorbic acid" refers to ascorbate reportedly consumed in the 24-hour dietary recall, without considering vitamin supplements.

The conclusions are complex and convoluted. They can be summarized by two large statements splashed in appropriate places in the original report.

> Among those who reported taking vitamin supplements, there is nothing to support any association between levels of ascorbic acid ingestion and periodontal health . . . Dental practitioners are better advised to concentrate on plaque control rather than vitamin C supplements to prevent and control periodontal disease in their patients.

This conclusion is in part the basis for the current recommendation of the Council on Dental Therapeutics of the American Dental Association.[4]

Is this the whole story?

By not including edulentous patients (those without teeth), did they not actually omit those with probably the worst periodontal disease? Would their findings have been different had they incorporated those with vitamin supplementation? What would have been the results had they included one or more of the biochemical measures of vitamin C state? Might there have been significant relationships between oral hygiene and the dietary conditions?

We'll look now into these and other questions.

Oral Hygiene: Playing With Words

As we have just learned, there is evidence that oral hygiene (however defined) is a significant factor in the genesis of periodontal pathosis. It seems also that different experts have their own definitions. Oral hygiene to some signifies the state of tooth cleanliness (how much junk is on the teeth?) to others the art of tooth cleansing (how well are you brushing your teeth?). By the way, junk on the teeth is variously labelled as calculus, tartar, plaque, debris, etc. Confusion stems from the common usage of the term "oral hygiene" which frequently doesn't recognize these differences. And so, things equal to the same thing become equal to each other. Therefore, it is generally held that there's a firm connection between how we clean our teeth and the amount of debris which accumulates around them.

In view of this chaos, we felt compelled to examine

the correlation of tooth cleansing and tooth cleanliness in the light of general body health.[5] Specifically, this interrelationship was viewed in terms of vitamin C level as measured by plasma ascorbic acid concentration. We tried and hopefully answered the following three questions.

1. To what extent does tooth cleanliness correlate with tooth cleansing? In other words, what's the connection between "oral debris" and "our toothbrushing habits?"

2. To what degree does tooth cleanliness correlate with one biochemical measure of health status, the plasma vitamin C level, regardless of tooth cleansing? Phrased differently, is there any correlation between the "plaque/calculus/tartar" and systemic health irrespective of "how we brush our teeth?"

3. Is the relationship between tooth cleansing and tooth cleanliness altered when viewed in the light of host state (plasma ascorbic acid level)? And so, is the "junk on your teeth" totally the result of "how much you brush?"

Two hundred middle income Caucasians participated in this study. Each subject was questioned regarding the frequency of toothbrushing. As a means of tooth cleanliness, a debris score was recorded. Incidentally, the examiner was unaware of the responses regarding brushing habits or plasma ascorbic acid findings.

With regard to the first question, Figure 9.1 shows

the frequency of daily toothbrushing on the horizontal axis and the mean debris scores on the vertical. The

Figure 9.1

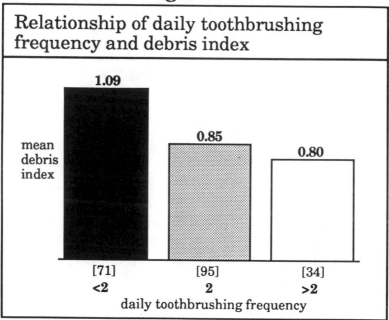

Relationship of daily toothbrushing frequency and debris index

group with the greatest toothbrushing (white column) shows the least debris. Hence, in answer to the first question, there does indeed appear to be a convincing relationship between tooth cleansing (toothbrushing frequency) and tooth cleanliness (debris score) irrespective of host state. And so, these observations are quite consistent with and support the current dental philosophy of the importance of local factors in periodontal health and sickness.

Apropos the second question, Figure 9.2 pictorially portrays the plasma ascorbic acid levels on the x-axis and the average debris scores on the ordinate. The data show that with the highest plasma vitamin C levels (white column), there is less tartar. Therefore, with-

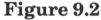

Figure 9.2

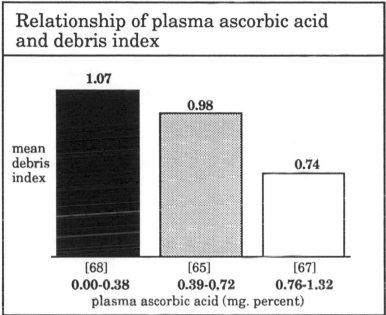

Relationship of plasma ascorbic acid
and debris index

mean debris index

1.07

0.98

0.74

[68]
0.00-0.38

[65]
0.39-0.72

[67]
0.76-1.32

plasma ascorbic acid (mg. percent)

in the limits of these data, there appears to be a very real correlation between vitamin C state and debris, irrespective of tooth cleansing habits.

Finally, the last question, Figure 9.3 shows the frequency of daily toothbrushing on the abscissa and the mean debris scores on the y-axis. Additionally, the 200 subjects were divided into two equal subgroups. The 100 subjects with the relatively poorer plasma ascorbic acid levels (less than 0.6 mg%) are shown by the black columns and the other 100 with the better vitamin C state (0.6+ mg%) by the white columns. Attention is directed to the fact that in those showing the lower plasma ascorbic acid scores, there is an obvious inverse relationship. In other words, the greater the tooth-brushing frequency, the less the debris (0.87). Interestingly, the data suggest that in those with relatively good ascorbate state (white columns) it's not too critical how frequently one brushes one's teeth!

Figure 9.3

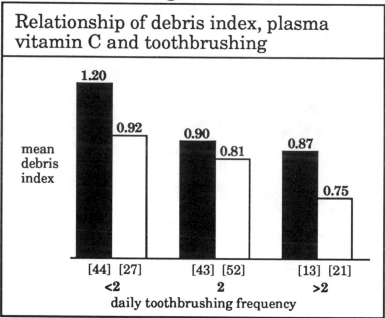

Relationship of debris index, plasma vitamin C and toothbrushing

This may be the explanation for the fact that some of us need to brush our teeth less than others.

The Flip Side of the Story

Historically, severe periodontal pathoses, including gingival hemorrhage, tooth mobility and loss of connective tissue attachment (which holds the teeth in their sockets) have been a classical clinical feature of ascorbic acid deficiency (Chapter Two). However, contemporary surveys, exemplified by the earlier two epidemiologic studies, suggest that the various forms of gingivitis and periodontitis result mainly from the activity of certain oral microorganisms that colonize the teeth and adjacent periodontal tissues. Even to many experts, periodontal disease is viewed as an infectious syndrome. (Our position on the role of microbes in health and sickness had been spelled out in Chapter Six.) Only a secondary, actually minor, role is postulated for ascorbate deficiency. According to official opinion, most of the epidemiological and experimental evidence accumulated during the past several decades has failed to demonstrate any significant **etiologic** relationship between vitamin C deficiency and the periodontal diseases.

Notwithstanding the orthodoxy, there are several score investigators who would disagree. For one, utilizing the now well-recognized ecologic formula (Chapter Five), we have examined the problem of prophylaxis (cleaning and polishing of the teeth) versus no prophylaxis in presumably healthy people with and without vitamin C supplementation.[6-8] In general, the evidence suggests that the cleaning and polishing of the teeth nets improvement in gingival inflammation.[6] The side of the mouth cleaned and polished resulted in a 30% improvement in gingivitis. Those treated with vitamin C without prophylaxis yielded a 45% reduction in gingival inflammation. Finally, with prophylaxis and ascorbate support, the figure climbed to 58% improvement. Who can argue that the ascorbates give us an added bonus? While the numbers for **sulcus depth**[7] and clinical tooth mobility[8] are different for obvious reasons, the patterns are all similar.

In all fairness, there are other well-designed studies. One is the work of Penelope Leggott and her associates at the University of California, San Francisco School of Dentistry and the U.S. Department of Agriculture Western Nutrition Research Center.[9]

Eleven healthy, nonsmoking men, aged 19 to 28, ate a rotating seven-day diet adequate in all nutrients except ascorbic acid. This basal diet, which contained less than five milligrams per day of AA, was supplemented with 60 mg/day for three weeks and zero mg/day for four weeks, 600 mg/day for three weeks and 0 mg/day for four weeks. Plasma, urine and leukocyte ascorbate levels, Plaque Index, Gingival Index, Bleeding Index and probing depths were monitored throughout the study. A uniform toothcleansing program was maintained in which instructions were reinforced biweekly.

Ascorbate concentrations in body fluids and leukocytes responded rapidly to changes in vitamin C intake. No **mucosal pathoses** or changes in plaque accumulation or probing depths were noted during any of the periods of depletion or supplementation. However, it cannot be too strongly mentioned that measures of gingival inflammation were directly related to the ascorbic acid status. The results suggest that the ascorbates may favorably influence early stages of gingivitis, particularly crevicular bleeding.

The Predictive Potential of C

While there continue to be many arguments about the role of vitamin C in health and sickness, one point is clear. Vitamin C can be used in the diagnosis and in the treatment of the suboptimal state.

What has not been mentioned is that hypoascorbemia also may serve in a predictive sense. There seems to be no argument but that seemingly similar persons treated seemingly similarly by similar or even the same practitioner may net different results. Some individuals show great improvement, others none, and some worsen. These people obviously aren't the same. The differences may be ascribed by playing with words such as resistance/susceptibility, tissue tolerance, immunity, or just great parents! The question for now is can one predict oral change by means of a study of vitamin C state?

To demonstrate the predictive potential, we'll employ the Lingual Ascorbic Acid Test (LAAT) discussed earlier (Chapter Four). Twenty-five presumably healthy subjects participated in an experiment to determine the predictive potential of an ascorbic acid measure in gingival state following oral prophylaxis.[10] The evidence suggests that the subjects with the better (shorter) lingual times have better gingiva prior to therapy. Further, the data indicate that better gingival results follow in subjects with better vitamin C state. Finally, the more restricted the ascorbate test range, the greater the predictiveness.

Table 9.1 summarizes the findings. It will be observed that 20 of the subjects (line 1) showed a LAAT of less than 35 seconds; 5 (line 2) greater than. Three points warrant special mention. It's interesting that the initial average gingival score for those with the better, the lower lingual scores (less than 35 seconds) is lower (0.90 versus 1.37). Second, this chart shows that three weeks after prophylaxis the mean gingival score is lower and therefore better, 0.58 (line 1) versus 1.22 (line 2) in those with the better vitamin C state. Thus, the gingival improvement is greater (36% versus 11%)

in the group with the more desired lingual scores.

Table 9.1

Changes in gingival state with oral prophylaxis on the basis of lingual vitamin C scores

lingual vitamin C test groups (seconds)	sample size	average gingival scores initial	final	% difference
<35	20	0.90	0.58	-36%
35+	5	1.37	1.22	-11%
<30	16	0.85	0.55	-35%
30+	9	1.25	1.00	-20%
<25	12	0.83	0.49	-41%
25+	13	1.15	0.91	-21%
<20	7	0.76	0.42	-45%
20+	18	1.08	0.82	-24%

Included are similar analyses for progressively more restricted LAAT ranges (e.g. less than 30 seconds, line 3, versus 30+ seconds, line 4; less than 25 seconds, line 5, versus 25+ seconds, line 6, etc.) The findings reported for the first groups are essentially the same.

It would appear that a tool, to be predictive, should meet three specifications. First, it should correlate with the parameter in question. Table 9.1 shows that this requirement is satisfied. Specifically, at the initial visit, the groups with the better (lower) gingival scores parallel the groups with the better (shorter) lingual times. Second, the instrument should forecast in advance of therapy the extent of change. Table 9.1 underlines this point; in each set of groups, those with the shorter (better) lingual time show greater percentage gingival improvement than the poorer vitamin-C groups. Finally, a tool gains in its predictive value if, as its range is restricted, its prognostication is enhanced. Table 9.1 emphasizes this to be the case. In the final groups, the subjects with lingual time less than 20 seconds (line 7) demonstrate the greatest improvement. The final average gingival score is lowest (closest to zero and, therefore, the best) of all categories (0.42) and the percentage improvement is the greatest (45%).

These findings are no accident. Similar conclusions were made from a subsequent study of the predictive potential of vitamin C state utilizing periodontal sulcus depth as the clinical indicator.[11]

Predictiveness for oral health/sickness is not the end of the story. We'll learn (Chapter Eleven) that the ascorbates are forecasters of longevity!

Summary and Conclusions

In May 1991, the Second World Congress on Vitamin C was held in San Diego. It provided the rare opportunity to examine the role of the ascorbates in stomatology.[12]

So, what transpired? *Vitamin C . . . who needs it?*

According to the information provided dealing with presumably healthy young people with the most minimal of periodontal pathosis, it would seem that everybody needs it.

What is not clear is how much. Certainly, providing these subjects with ten times the RDA (600 mg/day) produced favorable results. One must wonder whether the findings would not have been more dramatic had these subjects been studied with even larger amounts.

Skipping all of that, it's safe to say that the usual person with the average oral problems should fare better if vitamin C were added.

And there is another, hardly even mentioned bonus. The measurement of hypoascorbemia can be employed as a predictor of oral health even prior to dental treatment!

Thus far, the emphasis has been on so-called physical problems. Is it possible that there is also a body-mind connection? This will be our concern in the next chapter.

10

IT MAY NOT ALL BE IN YOUR HEAD!

The last chapter considered the tie-in of vitamin C and oral health. We emphasized the point that one of the earliest recognized findings in the scorbutic syndrome is bleeding and spongy gums.

Also suggested, though not particularly underlined, is that a second very prominent symptom is inordinate fatigability. Tiredness, under this and many other designations (exhaustion, weakness, burnout), is America's primary presenting complaint. This has been confirmed by a survey conducted under the auspices of the American Medical and Osteopathic Associations and sponsored by the Department of Health and Human Services.[1] In their study, a staggering 14 million Americans go to their doctors complaining of fatigue. Add to that uncounted millions who seek medical advice for other reasons but also mention significant exhaustion. Plus, millions more who never seek help but are nonetheless bushed all the time. In fact, America is being wiped-out by fatigue!

In many circles, it is viewed as a purely mental problem. More to the point, to be sure, there are many other symptoms and signs regarded as characteristic of mental and emotional stigmata. Depression heads the list and, in fact, is pictured as the common cold of mental disease. The historical record is clear that back in 1639, depression was recognized as a major component of scurvy during long sea voyages.

Is this the whole story?

Some experts would view these and other such nonspecific behavioral patterns as early mental symptomatology. Other authorities might well consider these findings purely and simply as subtle measures of the aging or aged state. This latter aspect and the role of vitamin C will be considered in Chapter Eleven.

Locking Up the Locked Up

What happens when one studies presumably healthy subjects from a penitentiary under carefully controlled metabolic conditions?

More to the point. Two investigators[2] tried to fill an obvious need from an experiment intended to provide systematic information on a broad range of human behavior during controlled ascorbic acid deprivation. Kinsman and Hood at the Metabolic Ward of the University of Iowa Medical Research Center studied five prisoners aged 26 to 52 for the better part of a year. The Psychological Screen (PS) was given near the beginning, middle and end of the depletion phase and at the midpoint of repletion. The PS measured four behavioral areas: mental functions, psychomotor performance, physical fitness and personality.

The venerable Minnesota Multiphasic Personality Inventory (MMPI) clearly showed that increased subjective reports of fatigue, lassitude, and depression became pronounced with ascorbic acid deficiency.

Detailed observations were made on the effects of behavior. In their own words, one of the conclusions was:

> The personality changes found to be associated with ascorbic acid deficiency correspond to the classical "neurotic triad" of the MMPI.

Robert Kinsman and James Hood have also provided us with more sophisticated confirmation of observations by others over many years.

Why hasn't such information been more available?

Is There a Stethoscope in the House?

This poignant question is actually the title of a most unusual report by Doctors McIntyre and Romano from the University of Rochester School of Medicine and Dentistry, New York.[3] It stems from two obvious contradictory facts. On the one hand, notwithstanding the palaver expressed in terms like psychosomatics, total body concepts, and mind-body wholeness, there still exists a body-mind separation. What happens in the usual doctor's office? More often than not, the physician makes an effort to explain the patient's problem on a physical basis. If this isn't possible, then he or she ascribes the condition to mental reasons. Psychotherapy follows.

So, here this. A survey was conducted in Rochester,

New York, of the attitudes and practices of psychiatrists (both in private practice and fulltime academic settings), psychiatric residents, internists, and fourth-year medical students concerning physical examinations of psychiatric patients. Only 13% of the psychiatrists frequently perform an initial physical examination on their inpatients; 8% often examined their outpatients. The largest number of psychiatrists report that they omit the physical exam because the patient has been referred to them after a physical examination by another physician or they refer the patient for such an appraisal. As but an aside, a notable percentage of psychiatrists in this sample report that they do not feel competent performing a physical examination.

Notwithstanding these devastating conclusions, what actually happens when conventional (meaning traditional and not necessarily adequate) physical exams are performed on routine so-called psychiatrically labelled subjects?

Richard Hall from the Medical College of Wisconsin at Milwaukee reported on his earlier studies at the University of Texas Medical School at Houston.[4] A survey of 658 consecutive psychiatric outpatients underwent physical examinations. Ten percent proved to have medical problems which could explain their psychiatric state. In a subsequent book "Psychiatric Presentations of Medical Illness,"[5] he says:

> The evidence is overwhelming that psychiatric symptoms frequently belie underlying medical illness. The incidence of such diseases producing psychiatric symptoms ranges from 5 to 42%, reflecting the population and selection variables employed.

Back to his original study. Hall and his cohorts

make the following observation:

> This study also demonstrated that a detailed medical review of systems, in combination with a careful physical examination and a . . . biochemical screen, would define the probable cause of psychiatric symptoms in 80% of cases where such disorders existed.

The actual numbers, the incidence and prevalence of a medical substrate in psychiatric disorders, can be argued. What is critical is that lots of patients deemed to be purely psychiatric when subjected to a somewhat-better physical examination (which incidentally doesn't include vitamin C studies), may have a medical basis for their behavioral problems.

Getting the Edge . . . Smart Drugs

Are behavioral problems exclusively confined to the domain of obviously sick mental patients? Clearly, there are other more subtle and possibly subversive aspects. How to classify forgetting where one puts one's glasses? Is forever losing keys a clue to mental illness? Should concentration fade with age? Can you improve your score on the next test?

These and other such queries have been and even more so are being addressed today. The speciality (not found in too many dictionaries) is termed noology. It comes from the Greek noos meaning mind and logos indicating discipline. Hence, for the purist, noology is defined as "the study of the mind, the science of phenomena regarded as purely mental in origin." The more practical approach is well-documented for the superscientists in the book by C. E. Giurgea.[6] Dean and Morgenthaler more palatably describe the public perception.[7]

There are many other books and even more periodical publications that serve as background material. What is most important is that these compounds are mind enhancers, cerebral achievers, or just plain "smart" agents. They may be nutrients . . . and interestingly vitamin C is one such nootropic preparation.

Early Cognitive Clues

Goodwin and his colleagues from the University of New Mexico (Albuquerque)[8] evaluated the association between nutritional status and cognitive functioning. In other words, they looked into the ability of the human to acquire, retain, and regurgitate information. The players comprised 260 well-educated and economically sound noninstitutionalized men and women older than 60 years who had no known physical illnesses and were receiving no medication. These individuals are usually regarded as well-nourished and therefore in perfect health. Nutritional status was evaluated by three-day food records and also by blood studies. Cognitive status was ascertained by two well-established and generally recognized psychometric tools. One is the Hallstead-Reitan Categories Test. This is a nonverbal automated procedure of abstract thinking and problem-solving ability, which is a sensitive indicator of minimal changes in mental status. The other is the Wechsler Memory Method. The interviewer reads a brief (one paragraph) story to each patient, and the subject is then asked to repeat the tale immediately. Thirty minutes later, the interviewee is again requested to recite the story.

There were a number of very exciting findings.

What is particularly relevant here is subjects with sub-optimal vitamin C blood levels scored worse on both tests. But let's be clear. Other nutrients not mentioned here also played a role.

Phrased in simple language, it's safe to conclude from these and many other studies that subclinical malnutrition is important in cognitive function. We will see (Chapter Eleven) that this phenomenon is especially prevalent in elderly individuals. Some have interpreted this discrepancy to suggest that most of the decrement in mental function reported with age isn't an inevitable age-caused event. Rather, these changes are secondary to various diseases and physical conditions that frequently accompany the geriatric experience. Let's get it straight. The purpose of this investigation by Goodwin and his group was to test the hypothesis that borderline or subclinical nutritional shortages might be associated with age-related cognitive deficiencies.

Precisely how significant these findings are in the usual scale of severity of mental complaints is still unsolved. What is abundantly clear is that there are possible vitamin C solutions to serious physiologic problems.

A Glimmer of Hope

Providing older people with extra vitamins sounds like a sensible course. Doctor James Goodwin (just cited) adds this:

> Studies in nursing homes have shown that when one provides half the residents a multivitamin and the other half a placebo (dummy pill), the staff will eventually be able to tell, with great accuracy, which half

was supplemented and which was not. The group on the vitamins is always doing better.

One of the nursing homes studied by Schorah (who has been mentioned several times before) and his cohorts [9] was a long-term care hospital in England. Incidentally, Schorah is with the Department of Chemical Pathology at the University of Leeds. They demonstrated that a supplement of vitamin C could, in many instances, help people who were so weak and listless to actually allow them to improve mentally and physically. The specifics of this trial included 115 men and women, age 59 to 97. Half of the subjects received a plain soft drink everyday and the other had the same beverage fortified with 1000 mgs of ascorbic acid. The experiment only lasted 28 days. The medical staff, not knowing which group was which, observed the patients to see whose appetite, interest in life around them, and general demeanor changed. As it turned out, in this short time frame, there was greater improvement in the supplemented group. On the average, they gained more weight and became more active. Some of the patients who had seemed beyond help surprised the staff with their recovery.

While this study was double-blind, it still was qualitative. To counter this point, we will now turn to an experiment of more quantitative design.

A Hard-to-Believe Look at the Common Mental Diseases

Anxiety and excitement have long been known to enhance the rate of breakdown of vitamin C. This point has been earlier developed (Chapter Seven) during the surgical experience. The process, it's suggested, may be exaggerated in schizophrenia by an abnormality of adrenaline metabolism.

Schizophrenics receiving the usual dietary ascorbate amounts are commonly found to be characterized by low blood vitamin C levels. As a matter of record, evidence of suboptimal blood vitamin C concentrations in most psychiatric patients has been gathered by a number of investigators over approximately 50 years. The following experiment was initiated in an attempt to clarify the possible role of vitamin C in such classical psychiatric situations.

Forty male patients participated in this experience.[10] Their mean age was 53 ranging from 29 to 59 and their average length of hospitalization was 18 years extending from 3 to 45. The principal diagnosis for the overwhelming number was schizophrenia. A pharmacist prepared two identical solutions, except that one contained ascorbic acid. The patients were prescribed one dose of the preparation daily for three weeks, those in the active group being given one gram of ascorbic acid per day. Before and after the trial, all the subjects were examined for scorbutic stigmata, along with an assessment of hemaglobin and blood and urine vitamin C measurements.

In order to assess psychologic state, the depression scale of the Minnesota Multiphasic Personality Inventory (MMPI) was included. This, as we already know, is probably the most popular self-rating questionnaire but obviously provides only subjective interpretation. Secondly, the highly-celebrated Wittenborn Psychiatric Rating Scales (WPRS) were used as a measure of overtly observable behavior in the patient made possible by both the doctor and the ward nurse.

Clearly, the latter provided a more objective estimate of the patient's condition. Both of these scales were performed before and after the trial.

The results, observed by G. Milner at the Tower Hospital in Leicester, are clear. With the patients self-rating scoring system (MMPI), there was a statistically convincing improvement in the depression scale. Of the six categories of the Wittenborn, there were three sub-scales (manic, depression, and paranoid state) that were clearly significantly improved.

This fascinating story is one of a reasonably well-controlled blind trial of ascorbic acid versus placebo saturation. Standardized objective and subjective psychologic testing was employed to assess changes dependent upon AA consumption. Hypoascorbemia was found. It is reasonable to conclude that mentally disturbed subjects are shown to have an unusually high demand for vitamin C. Unequivocal mitigation in the depressive, manic, and paranoid symptomatology resulted together with an improvement in overall personality functioning following fortification with one gram of the ascorbates. Finally, the bottom line is that chronic emotionally-laden subjects would be well-served by the administration of vitamin C.

Now to the other big mental problem . . . manic depressive state. The effect of vitamin C in these syndromes was assessed by a double-blind placebo controlled, crossover trial. This was part of a series of studies based on the assumption that heavy metals (and particularly vanadium) may be a contributing factor to such disorders. Twenty-four (twelve manic and twelve depressed) subjects participated in this study by Naylor and Smith at The University of Dundee in Great Britain.[11] Each patient completed two generally accepted psychometric tests for the assessment of the manic/depressive state. Immediately thereafter, each subject was provided with either a three gram ascorbic acid effervescent tablet dissolved in water or a placebo which was a similar looking tablet with a like taste and appearance. They were rated hourly by these psychometric tests. The following day the procedure was reversed.

The most exciting observation is that in the vitamin treated group, the severity was reduced within the first hour and then declined even more rapidly between the second and fourth hours. The point of the matter is that whether manic or depressed, a single three gram dose of ascorbic acid significantly altered the clinical state in a matter of hours!

Beyond Talk Therapy

There was a time (and not too long ago) when going to a psychiatrist meant lying on a couch and just talking. This was the era of Sigmund Freud and his followers (e.g. Jung, Adler, and Horney) and even some of their disciples.

Today, there is still, but much less, talk. What's more fashionable is the use of drugs in the management of emotionally-disturbed people.

Just for kicks, get yourself an insert from almost any common packaged drug. You'll find a section marked "indications" intended to provide the reader with the justifications for that particular agent. We'll call it a "plus." There'll also be a section marked "contraindications" which outlines the undesirableness of the substance . . . why, in fact, we ought not to use this drug. Think of this as a "minus." Then there are sections "precautions," "warnings," "adverse effects," "overdosage" which are nothing more than polite synonyms and therefore more minuses.

Table 10.1 summarizes six commonly employed psychotherapeutic prescription drugs.[12] You'll note that with remarkable regularity, there are a small number of indications. For the entire group there are 128. You may wish to think of them as "benefits." On the other hand, overall, there are approximately 2245 minuses.

Table 10.1

Reasons for and against common psychotherapeutic drugs expressed by lines of text in insert		
drugs	**pluses**	**minuses**
Valium	19	114
Xanax	60	581
Prozac	22	597
Haldol	15	443
Halcion	9	271
Elavil	3	239

These are the undesirable "risks." For the entire group, there appears to be 18 times more minus points than favorable ones. And, there are other issues:

• The most recent figures from the Centers for Disease Control suggest that 2.1 to 2.6% of the adult population can be regarded as suffering with "serious mental illness (SMI)."[13]

• In America, one woman in five and one man in seven take the tranquilizer Valium at a cost of approximately 60¢ a pill.

• In 1990, over two billion dollars was spent for psychotherapeutic agents. This trans lates to $8.01 for every living man, woman and child.

Obviously, psychotherapeutic drugs have their place but should be viewed cautiously in terms of benefits versus risks. Where does vitamin C fit into this picture?

J. Jancar, from the Stokes Park Hospital in Bristol reported the results of the first two years of a tranquilizer-withdrawal scheme, which consisted of three months of the gradual elimination of tranquilizers and their replacement—tablet for tablet—by ascorbic acid.[14] This was followed by three months of gradual withdrawal of vitamin C and 18 months observation of the patients.

What makes this study exciting is its double blind nature; only the pharmacist, another consultant and the author were aware of the actual ingredient. A hospital was selected which housed severely mentally retarded males, mostly middle aged and elderly, and included fifty-seven patients who were already on psychotherapeutic substances. The length of treatment with various tranquilizing agents, before the trial, varied from four months to thirteen years and eight months. At the end of the two year experiment, thirty (53%) of the fifty-seven patients on pretrial tranquilizers no longer required these substances. The added benefit should be emphasized that there were also no side effects. This is heightened by the evidence (Table 10.1) of the usual problems with standard tranquilizing substances.

In the light of these (and other) studies, it would seem that the ascorbates ought to receive more serious attention as alternatives to some of our current psychotherapeutic agents.

Summary and Conclusions

In recent years, there has been an increasing awareness that the body/mind dichotomy is unreal. Notwithstanding, the usual sequence of events is to look for a physical accounting of the patients' problems. When no such diagnosis is forthcoming, the tendency then is to ascribe by exclusion a mental (emotional, behavioral) conclusion. It would seem that one explanation, is that presumably the practitioner is so skilled that if he/she cannot find a physical basis for the patient's complaints, then the problem must be in the mind!

In this chapter, we have presented evidence, sometimes qualitative and sometimes measured. In any case, ascorbic acid (as well as other nutrients) plays a causative role in behavior. This may be reflected in minor mental changes, ranging from its earliest subtle expressions (as in the aging subject) to its role in clearcut and obvious psychiatric symptomatology.

And so, *Vitamin C . . . who needs it?* It would seem that those with obvious psychiatric manifestations ought to consider the ascorbates as part of their therapeutic armamentarium. At least, it should be viewed as an alternative to the present state of affairs. At the moment, 46% of serious mental illness (SMI) patients take at least one prescription drug for their mental problem; 25% take two.[13] There's reasonable evidence to suggest that those with seemingly minor mental problems, in the fuzzy area, might also fare more successfully with such supplementation.

We have been examining, albeit in a very arbitrary fashion, the role of vitamin C in many different and diverse syndromes. In the final analysis, the mother of all disease patterns is the aging and the aged state. This will be the theme of the next chapter.

11

CAN WE CHANGE
THE HUMAN CLOCK?

There is a lot of interest in the aging process and the aged state. Perhaps the most compelling fact is that more and more people are living into the golden years. The record shows that at the turn of this century in the USA, one person in 25 was over the age of 65. By the year 2000, it will change to one in five. In other words, we've climbed from 4 to 20%, a fivefold increase. And all this has happened in the last 100 years.

It therefore isn't surprising that with such burgeoning numbers have come several myths and magics.

The first follows in response to the question, "To what do you attribute your long life?" The reply more often than not is "I chose good parents." Implied is that genetics is central to long life. No question. There is indeed an ongoing still-unresolved nature (genetics) versus nurture (environment) debate.[1] While inheritance certainly plays an undeniable role in health/sickness, from a practical standpoint the environment is probably more important. (Unlike genetics, you can do something about it!)

The next fiction is that the aging process moves along a well-defined path with distinct markers. This is evident by such a cliche as "What do you expect for your age?" The public and the professions have it in their heads that at a certain time the blood cholesterol should be higher, the number of wrinkles should be set, and it's perfectly alright to begin to forget where one puts one's glasses. Not true. As a matter of fact, we have already discussed this subject as it relates to blood sugar (Chapter Eight). Some of us (unfortunately too many) seem older than our years. Occasionally (rarely but fortunately) there are those who look younger.

Actually, When Does Old Age Begin?

There is another myth. We assume that elderly problems are confined to the elderly years. Not true. For one, there's ample evidence that approximately 90% of young and healthy American soldiers killed in combat in Korea showed on autopsy evidence of hardening of the arteries at the tender age of 20. Is this generally-recognized sign of old age true of all youngsters? Autopsies of like-aged Korean soldiers wiped-out in the very same combat showed only that 10% had arteriosclerosis. So, it seems as if this picture of the aging state is "made-in-America" (actually in western and highly developed societies).

Is there more?

How about the observations of toddlers who meet an untimely death (i.e. crawl into a refrigerator and close the door or climb into a tub and scald themselves to death)? Autopsies in such instances already disclose the ravages of hardening of the arteries. These bits of clearcut information suggest that likely the so-called geriatric problems begin, in fact, during the pediatric years!

How Does the Aging Process Start?

Cited already are the infinite gradations from white to black. At one end is perfect (pure) health. At the other pole are all of the serious and significant illnesses.

What is dominant is the cellular tug-of-war. We have already, on numerous occasions, made mention of the constant and relentless forces which invite malfunction and death at the cellular level. For example, now we know that each puff on a cigarette contains 10^{14} free radical in the tar phase and 10^{15} in the gas phase.[2] In parallel are those positive vectors designed to maintain stability and health. This, in fact, is the basis for the free-radical hypothesis of illness.

The critical factors are the intensity and the duration of these counter energies. In the case of the blahs or the common cold, the vectors are of low intensity and of short duration. When these elements endure and become of greater amplitude, then the more serious killing and crippling syndromes appear.

The myth is that old age does all this. Richard Young from the University of California in Los Angeles has provided the best and most succinct response:[3]

> Age (as a cause) can be discounted . . . because time is a dimension, not a causal factor. The challenge is to identify the factors that are active during the pas-

sage of time.

Phrased another way, age is not a risk factor. It only provides the time necessary for risk forces to play havoc.

When a person ages, these same oxidative processes are working at a low intensity over a long period of time.

Recent evidence shows that this process can be slowed or halted by antioxidants.[4, 5, 6] Hence for our purposes, the burning question here is, "What does vitamin C have to do with altering the human timepiece?"

Changing the Human Clock

What is it that can be altered?

The answer to this question requires critical definition. Specifically, what do we mean by life span and life expectancy? On the one hand, life span represents the biologic limits of living. In other words, it poses the question as to when the human parts just break down and make life no longer possible. It's been said that Methuselah made it to 969 years! The Scriptures (Genesis 6:3) hint, if they don't promise, 120 healthy and happy years. Moses is said to have lived 12 decades (and believe it or not without eyeglasses). Interestingly, many distinguished scientists in longevity research also argue that the human organism should endure for this timespan. The most compelling logic for this hypothesis is that all wild animals including man are known to live ten times puberty. Recognizing puberty at approximately twelve years, it figures that the human organism should also make it for about 120 years.

As one might expect, these estimates aren't all that clearcut. There are equally celebrated investigators who argue for other numbers.

Interestingly, well-documented human survival curves by decades since 1900 converge at the same time showing the maximum survival age seems to be fixed at approximately 85 to 100 years.

How well is Mr. America doing?

In 1900 the life expectancy was 47 years. This will be approximately 74 years in 2000. So, unlike life span, life expectancy can and has been significantly extended.

Life expectancy figures are available for approximately 160 countries around the world. In early 1990, the Centers for Disease Control released statistics showing that the US ranks 17th in life expectancy among the 33 "developed" countries (incidentally, Japan is tops and Switzerland is right behind).

Hence, as far as the quantity of life goes, we are obviously not doing too well.

How Much Life Could There Be?

As limited as our information seems to be, we have some quantitative data that tells us something about the quality and quantity of life based on health practices.

Many investigators and clinics have tried to sort out lifestyle. The Human Population Laboratory (HPL)[7] has concluded that, of the many different characteristics of lifestyle, seven provide a reasonably accurate and predictable profile. They are smoking, weight in relation to desirable standards for height, drinking (alcohol), hours of sleep, regularity of meals, eating breakfast and physical activity.

Incidentally, in a later report,[8] the HPL confirmed that only five health practices (excluding regularity of

Table 11.1

Average remaining lifetime using death rates of three health practice groups and California life-table, 1959-1961

sex	age	health practices			California
		0-3	4-5	6-7	1959-1961
men	45	22	28	33	28
	55	14	20	25	20
	65	11	14	17	13
	75	7	10	11	8
	85	7	6	5	5
	90	3	3	3	
women	45	39	34	36	33
	55	20	25	28	25
	65	12	17	20	17
	75	9	12	13	10
	85	5	8	8	5
	90	3	4	5	

meals and eating breakfast) provide adequate prediction.

That the original combination is quite predictive is demonstrated in Table 11.1. According to the California Abridged Life Tables (1959-1961), the average 45-year-old male (irrespective of his lifestyle) will live 28 more years (line 1). In other words, the life expectancy of the on-the-street California male 45 years old is 73. If this individual engages in zero to three of the just-mentioned health practices, he can be expected to only live

22 more years. Should one participate in four or five of such health variables, the expectancy is increased 28 years. Finally, the addition of six or seven of the desirable lifestyles makes it possible to extend life until 78 years of age. We see here that there's a very definite relationship between health benefits (as arbitrary as they are) and length of life. Such predictions can be made for both men and women at different ages (lines 2-12).

Can we sharpen our predictions? What would happen if we correlated life expectancy based on one or more specific dietary characteristics?

Does anybody have information that contributes directly or otherwise to this question?

James E. Enstrom, an epidemiologist at the University of California in Los Angeles looked at this very problem.[9] He analyzed a federal government survey of 11,348 adults ages 25 to 74 who were examined during 1971-1974 and followed through 1984. People with intakes of about 300 to 400 mgs of vitamin C daily, roughly half from food, were compared with those who got less than 50 mgs daily. The findings were adjusted for age, sex, race, smoking, disease history and other differences.

Conclusions are clear. Men consuming 300 to 400 mgs per day showed an overall mortality reduction of 42%. Translated into life expectancy, this suggests an added longevity of six years!

He also found a 10% lower overall death rate— equivalent to one extra year of life—among women who consumed a few hundred milligrams of vitamin C. More specifically, the improvements seem to be in mortality due to heart disease and cancer.

Obviously, the final chapter hasn't been written.

More needs to be done. However, it is noteworthy that the amounts of ascorbic acid which showed these unusual benefits were the very same quantities earlier reported (Chapter Three) for the "ideal" person!

The Predictive Potential Revisited

Aside from the diagnostic and therapeutic implications of ascorbate testing, we have also alluded to its predictive role. Doctor T. S. Wilson and his group at the Barncoose Hospital in Cornwall, England[10] carried out a highly innovative experiment. It consisted of a study of 159 patients admitted to an acute geriatric unit in 1968 in which ordinarily one out of three subjects expires within the first four weeks. On the one hand, he studied the subjects with relatively poor vitamin C state (less than 12 mcg%) as measured in the buffy coat layer of the blood. (The significance of this level of vitamin C has been discussed in some detail in Chapter Four.) The other subset was slightly less hypoascorbemic (12+ mcg%). Lo and behold, the mortality within the first four weeks was significantly less in those with the relatively better blood vitamin C picture.

As incomplete as these data are, they do tend to corroborate the earlier work from the Human Population Laboratory. They also make one wonder how much more sophisticated our predictions would be if such avenues were pursued and refined.

The Good Life?

Enough about life extension. Surely, what we all really want is to add life to our years . . . rather than

just years to life.
Did you know:

• every day 4,000 Americans suffer a heart attack?

• one out of ten Americans, during their lifetime, will have a nervous breakdown?

• by the time we are 40, 25% of us have no teeth?

• everyone sooner or later seems to need eyeglasses?

• two out of three families will feel the pain of cancer?

• it's estimated that 36,000,000 Americans from toddlers to centenarians suffer from some kind of arthritis?

From these nontrivia, it is clear that, as we grow older, most if not all of us progressively lose our organs so that, in fact, we really don't die . . . we simply run out of parts! This can hardly be called good quality of life. What should happen (and certainly does in wild animals) is to function optimally up to a point, hopefully go to sleep, and simply not wake up. Or at least to have a catastrophic experience like a sudden massive heart attack or stroke and in seconds or minutes expire.

In short, modern medicine hasn't made it possible to live as long and as well as we should.

And so, the next question is, "Is there a demonstrated role for vitamin C in the quality of life?" To the extent possible here's a reasonably well-controlled experiment on its effect.

A Not-Too-Generally Known Benefit for Old People

C. J. Schorah and his colleagues at the General Infirmary in Leeds (U.K.) conducted a double-blind controlled prospective trial.[11] The specifics included one gram ascorbate per day versus placebo supplementation. The patient sample consisted of 94 elderly long-term geriatric in-house subjects. They characteristically had low initial plasma and leukocyte ascorbic acid levels (mean 0.17 mg/100 ml plasma and 10.1 mcg leukocytes). After only two months of treatment, both plasma and white cell levels had increased substantially only in those receiving vitamin C supplements. And in this group, there were also slight but significant rises in the mean body weight (0.41 kg), in blood protein levels, and improvement in capillary health (reduction in purpura and petechial hemorrhages). Finally, in the placebo group, not only was there not any improvement, but actually a worsening of these same parameters.

In other words, just about every biochemical and clinical characteristic studied indicated that these not-very-high doses of ascorbate netted a better quality of life in this group of elderly.

70 Going on 40 Biochemically?

We earlier asked the question, "Can one sharpen

one's prediction?" Resoundingly yes. In the real world, can one turn matters around and actually make people biochemically younger?

Eric Bowers and Michael Kubik studied 50 elderly people (mean age 76) living at home in the industrial midlands of England.[12] They found an average plasma ascorbic acid level of only 0.23 mg/100 ml and a mean white blood cell level of 12.3 mcg. They were compared to 200 young people (average age 35) with a mean plasma level of 0.78 mg/100 ml and an average leucocyte concentration of 26 mcg. These hospital consultants reported that white blood cell ascorbic acid levels in their elderly subjects could be raised, in two weeks, to the same levels as in the young people by giving them 120 mg of vitamin C daily.

Helen Newton and her colleagues from the University of Leeds (England) also examined the phenomenon of "making people younger."[13] Their study differed from that of Bowers and Kubik in a number of ways. First, this study took place 20 years later. Second, these British investigators utilized hospital instead of ambulatory subjects who were obviously sicker. Next, this experiment not only included the administration of the ascorbates but the double-blind design with placebo as part of the picture. Fourth, the evidence suggested not only that elderly people could be made biochemically younger but also even younger than the young subjects.

It is fascinating to note that the supplementation was even smaller than that in the earlier study. Actually, the amounts in this report were 30 to 50 mg in one experiment and 100 mg in another. Finally, and most importantly, in both of these trials, it is convincingly demonstrated that one can biochemically rejuvenate elderly subjects in a relatively short period of time with ascorbate supplementation.

At the risk of oversimplification, what we discover is that one can, in effect, significantly reverse the (biochemical) age!

Summary and Conclusions

There's enough data to suggest that those of us living in civilized societies aren't doing as well as we could or should.

The good news is that the evidences of old age like hardening of the arteries can actually be slowed, stopped, and even reversed by relatively simple lifestyle changes.

In this chapter, we have had the opportunity to witness improvement in the quantity and quality of life under reasonably supervised conditions with the simple administration of the ascorbates. So, *Vitamin C . . . who needs it?* It would seem wise that, across the board, elderly people could profit by additional vitamin C supplementation.

What next . . . we'll try, in the forthcoming chapter, to sum up the relationship of vitamin C in other not-well-known experiments utilizing the skin as the centerpiece for discussion.

12

THE SKIN: OTHER EXTRAORDINARY CONNECTIONS!

For the past few chapters, we've been wrestling with a collection of published (but still-not-well-known) carefully-executed experiments. From these, one must conclude that vitamin C has great versatility. It almost seems to be the perfect panacea.

Have we, in fact, captured the complete picture? Hardly.

If our purpose is to present the total story, then we've only just begun. But our aim continues to be simply to convey representative answers to the question, *Vitamin C . . . who needs it?*

What we'll do in this chapter is to attempt to wrap up the story utilizing the human coat as our common denominator. Why the skin?

- It is, by all authorities, the largest organ of the body.

• The surface layer, because of its obvious visibility, makes it more available for examination and manipulation (e. g. biopsy).

• The integument (skin) serves as the major interface between the internal and external worlds.

• The cutaneous tissues serve many critical functions notably of a protective nature.

In addition to these listed nontrivia, the dermal layers are the venue of many problems.

• Some 30% of Americans have dermatologic conditions requiring a physician's service.

• During World War II, there were more evacuations from the South Pacific theater for skin diseases than for battle casualties.

In the light of its many functions and the almost epidemic nature of its problems, it should come as no surprise that skin coat care is costly.

• In some parts of the USA, acute and chronic diseases of the skin account for over half of all workmen's compensation cases.

• It is estimated that more than $3 billion, which boils down to $12 for every man, woman and child, was spent in 1982 for physician services, hospitalizations and drugs for skin conditions.

For these reasons and others, the skin is the most unique of our organs.

• The psychologic role this envelope and its appendages, the hair and nails, plays in our appearance can't be overestimated.

• $400 million was expended in 1982 only for topical over-the-counter preparations.

But more about this point later.

Shooting C

We earlier made mention that one of the most unique features of our dermal envelope is that it readily lends itself to measurement (i.e. tourniquet test). For the record, there's a not-too-well-known intradermal vitamin C test reported elsewhere (Chapters One and Four). Dunbar and his University of Alabama Medical Center team performed this particular cutaneous technique on 16 presumably healthy dental students under fasting conditions.[1] One thousand milligrams of ascorbic acid was then administered intravenously (IV) to each of these subjects. The intradermal time values, expressed in minutes, were then redetermined at 15 minutes, 24 and 48 hours after the injection.

To better understand the findings, it must be remembered that, as the tissue ascorbate increases, the intradermal time diminishes. Figure 12.1 represents the average intradermal response of the 16 dental students. Under fasting conditions, the mean intradermal score is 24 minutes. Within 15 minutes, after the IV injection of one gram of AA, the tissue time decreased to 12 (actually cut in half). Subsequent analyses 24 and 48 hours later revealed a return to almost the original state.

Figure 12.1

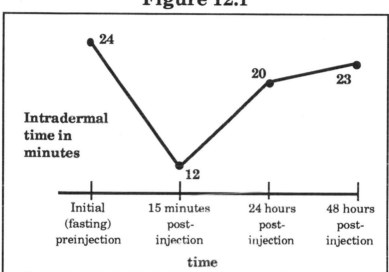

The important point to be gleaned from this simple experiment is that integumentary vitamin C can be measured. Secondly, one can pack a significant amount of ascorbic acid into the skin in minutes. Finally, this intravenous shock, as it were, lasts for hours as shown by a return to the original scores in approximately two days.

The Human Thermostat

In Chapter Five, we made the point that one of the

exciting actions of the ascorbates was in the critical area of thermoregulation. We summarized our findings on this very subject back in 1982.[2]

Sometimes technology takes its toll. In really hot climates, the parking lot of a shopping mall can be the hard bed for unconscious bodies of people who couldn't quite make it from the air-conditioned car to the cool supermarket or back.

The Hot News

Workers in America's southland may have it rough, but South African mines provide a far more dramatic working climate. Mine owners long ago learned to initiate all sorts of acclimatization procedures in step-by-step progression. Even so, the rookies on the job suffer severely from the heat.

Researchers from the Industrial Hygiene Division of the Chamber of Mines of South Africa, led by N. B. Strydom, divided sixty new mine workers into three groups.[3] The first subset received 250 mg of C per day. The second group was administered 500 mg daily. Lastly, there were those who took a dummy tablet (placebo). All the men then went through the progressive stages of acclimatization in chambers simulating a mine's atmosphere. Various measurements of heat adaptation (temperature, heart rate, amount of perspiration) were recorded.

Both AA groups showed a clear advantage. For example, rectal temperatures were taken at 0, 1, 2, 3 and 4 hours after exercise each day. The ascorbate groups "won" by 24 hours on the average. And a startling 35% of those "winners" adapted in only three or four days. Some (on the placebo) unhappily even failed the ten day test!

The Not-so-Hot News

Early research on rats and guinea pigs showed that high levels of vitamin C can counteract cold temperature states. A group of monkeys given 325 mg of ascorbic acid before being exposed to subfreezing temperatures fared far better than the lower animals administered only 25 mg daily.

Thus, human beings bound for snow might want to think not only of warm pants but also of popping about 4000 mg of vitamin C per day. That's the human equivalent (given 150 pounds of weight) of the amount provided the monkeys.

Professor M. Nakamura and co-workers from the Faculty of Medicine, Hirosake University in Japan,[4] decided to enlist some volunteers on the theory that what's good for monkeys is good for medical students. They administered 200 mg of ascorbic acid daily for 17 days to 20 healthy young adults whose diets furnished about 80 mg of vitamin C each day of the testing period. By measuring skin temperature before and 40 minutes after exposure to cold (5°C or 41°F), the investigators conclusively showed that the C-supplemented subjects demonstrated higher skin temperatures.

And Then There's Also the Itchy Evidence

To the nonsufferer, pruritus (prickly heat) sounds like an innocuous enough little ailment. But the tiny pimples can close pores, causing an abrupt elevation of body temperature. Moreover, the intense itching and sensations of "crawlies" and burning can interfere with sleep and concentration. Secondary infection is common when victims scratch themselves. So, this could all make for a serious problem.

What is the connection between vitamin C and prickly heat?

Doctor T. C. Hindson was first drawn to ascorbic acid as a treatment for pruritus while he served as a dermatologist at the British Military Hospital in Singapore.[5] Here again we learn of another happy accidental finding. (You may recall we have earlier discussed serendipity.) He interviewed an Australian Air Force officer who had suffered severe heat rash in the groin area. There had been scratching, provoking a secondary infection. (Medical diagnosis: intertriginous dermatitis secondarily infected with monilia.) The painful rash had lasted for a year, resisting all forms of therapy. Then the officer caught a cold (as the saying goes) and on his own, took one gram of vitamin C each day for a week. Lo and behold, his heat rash cleared up. On this wise hunch, Doctor Hindson placed the patient on 1000 mg of ascorbic acid as the sole treatment for the dermatologic condition. Just ten days later, examination showed a normal groin area.

Hindson decided to enlarge this experiment—first with five children given vitamin C in amounts equivalent to the milligrams per body weight of the Air Force officer.[5] He then worked with 30 kids who had suffered repeated attacks of heat rash. Of the fifteen youngsters given ascorbic acid for two weeks, fourteen were entirely rash free or improved. Of the fifteenchildren provided dummy pills, only four kids showed any resolution. For the next two months, all thirty were administered vitamin C and the story ends happily . . . no further rash was noted in any of the children!

The report continues with Hindson working with an associate at the hospital. They used plastic bandages to wrap one arm each of 36 apparently healthy servicemen for 48 hours.[6] Vitamin C (one gram daily) was given to 18 subjects, and a placebo to the other 18. One week after the arms were unwrapped, 17 placebo subjects still showed sweat gland fatigue (hypohidrosis), 10 of them markedly. But, in the ascorbic acid group only two subjects showed hypohidrosis—and then only to a mild degree.

The New NonScreen Sunscreen

Solar radiation contributes to a variety of cutaneous (and even systemic) biologic effects which may be both useful and harmful.[7-8] There's no question but that exposure to small amounts of radiation in the ultraviolet (UV) range is a requirement for the vital vitamin D photosynthesis in the skin. This is the good news.

There is also no argument that larger exposures may yield the positive (highly desirable cosmetic) and negative (pain, burning) effects of sunburn. And so, the cardinal question is how to get the most benefits from the sun with the least damage?

The conventional approach is the use of sunscreens. The most popular are topical agents in the form of solutions, gels, creams or ointments. The central ingredient is generally a vitamin, paraaminobenzoic acid (PABA) and its derivatives. But, unfortunately, there is increasing evidence that these common and conventional sunscreens may interfere with vitamin D synthesis. In other words, the situation is one where our greatest protection against the sun is made possible by means of a vitamin (PABA) which, in turn, interferes with the formation of still another vitamin (D).

And so, is it possible to provide the sunscreen effect by other means? It now looks like a different vitamin (C) may be the answer.

A group at Duke University has shown significant UV protection to pig skin by topical applications of the ascorbates.[9] It logically followed to test this out in the human.[10] To do this, ten volunteers were pretreated for five days on their **volar** forearms with a 10% l-ascorbic acid solution or an indistinguishable placebo, then irradiated with UV. At 24 hours, both arms were photographed using color slides. The films were then analyzed for erythema (redness) effect. By careful measurement, only the sites treated with topical vitamin C showed a 22% significant reduction of redness. Even simple inspection confirmed the protective effect of the ascorbates.

We've had frequent opportunities to mention vitamin C and the free radical hypothesis. Once again, it is well to emphasize the story. Simple sunburn is an excellent example of the ravages of oxidative damage. The ascorbates in the form of an ointment provide a superb illustration of the protective effects of a powerful antioxidant.

... And There's Another Wrinkle

If only we had looked back into the past and listened to history! In Chapter Five, we learned of the versatility of the ascorbates. Clearly the health of the connective tissues is very much at the mercy of vitamin C. This is consistent with the general knowledge that

AA works by nourishing fibroblasts, the cells that produce skin-boosting collagen. Here is more proof that this fits with the obvious that smoother skin on top means better subcutaneous collagen support.

There are interesting connections between lifestyle and skin health. We have mentioned in earlier chapters the devastating effects of recreational drugs like tobacco upon ascorbic acid metabolism. Not previously cited is the study by H. W. Daniell, M.D. of 1104 subjects.[11] The severity of facial wrinkles correlated with a history of habitual cigarette smoking even after adjustment for age and outdoor exposure. The relationship between tobacco intake and wrinkling was striking in both sexes soon after the age of 30. It was certainly related to the duration and intensity of tobacco usage. Smokers in the 40- to 49-year age group were as likely to be prominently wrinkled as nonsmokers who were 20 years older! In effect, this may well be one of the reasons why so many people are biochemically 40 going on 70 (Chapter 11).

What happens when one puts these pieces of the puzzle together? A vitamin C cream may soon give Retin-A a run for its money. A new C-based wrinkle-reducer already has been tested on several hundred people, including fifty at the University of Wisconsin-Madison by Lorraine Meisner, Ph.D, in the Department of Preventive Medicine.[12] What is most intriguing is that approximately 95% reported a reduction in wrinkling within six weeks to two months. And even more comforting is the fact that the C-treatment appears to be without side effects (which is certainly not the case with Retin-A).

Summary and Conclusions

This chapter provides us with an extraordinary opportunity to summarize experimental evidence from reasonably well-designed and supervised vitamin C studies.

We have here the unusual opportunity of reminding ourselves that the skin is a superb mirror of wellness and ill-health. Let's not forget the importance of the not-too-well-known but reasonably accurate intradermal test cited earlier (Chapter Four).

Thirdly, in Chapter Five we reviewed some of the many and diverse functions of the ascorbates. Evidence to confirm these has now once again been provided by experiments with thermoregulation, collagen synthesis, and free radical damage.

Up to this point, the use of ascorbic acid has been emphasized largely by oral administration, and parenterally (mostly intravenously). Now we learn that vitamin C can serve a potentially useful purpose by inunction (applied to the skin). Incidentally, we'll also discover in the next chapter its use in the form of eyedrops.

The information in this chapter is obvious and reasonable. If true, then there's a paradox. We have examined five of the current leading dermatology textbooks.[13-17] Would you believe that not a word appears regarding the role of vitamin C in skin and health disease!

Until now in this monograph, the studies described have met the most rigid criteria for experimental design. There are other interesting and informative projects that, for all kinds of reasons, can't or don't meet these strict standards. Such studies will be emphasized in the next chapter.

13

VITAMIN C ... WHO ELSE MIGHT NEED IT?

What we have been doing is, in effect, splicing together a story based on the most sophisticated available data. We've been examining vitamin C under controlled experimental conditions. All of the rest of the evidence, the not-so-hard proof, remains on the cutting floor. Before we discard this material, we ought to examine it with the understanding that, while the proof is not complete, it is worthy of some scrutiny. Hence, the purpose of this chapter is to review the not-so-perfect experimentation as it relates to the question, *Vitamin C ... who needs it?*

The Classical Epidemiologic Tool

A review of the literature quickly discloses that the overwhelming body of fact about the ascorbates in health and sickness is correlative and derived by epidemiologic techniques.

A characteristic analysis of one such survey has been carried out by A. J. Verlangieri and his colleagues from the University of Mississippi.[1] The report was prompted by the generally-agreed-upon observation of the recent decline (1964-1978) in cardiovascular mortality in the United States. Further, there was the suggestion that these death patterns might be related in some way to the consumption of fruits and vegetables during that same time frame. This study tested the hypothesis that increased consumption of these fresh foods had a protective effect against cardiovascular mortality among the American population during these 15 years. It further suggests this effect may be due to their vitamin C content.

On the one hand, consumption tables were utilized to ascertain the ascorbic acid content in the foods and the rate of intake over time on the natural history of cardiovascular diseases. It was calculated from production data by the Economics, Statistics, and Cooperative Services and the Science and Education Administration of the Consumer and Food Economics Institute.

Independently, the mortality by cause of death statistics were computed in accordance with the World Health Organization's (WHO) regulations using the *International Classification of Diseases* (ICD).

Interestingly, these investigators employed two generally-held noncardiovascular disorders (diabetes mellitus and cystic fibrosis) as controls.

Cited directly from their report:

> From the analyses of data collected in this study, the investigators conclude that the consumption of fruits and vegetables, particularly those that are rich

sources of vitamin C, may offer some protection against cardiovascular disease mortality.

This well-designed and carefully-executed study at least confirms what has already been cited (Chapter Seven) in carefully-controlled and under double-blind conditions.

Eat Your Way Out of High Blood Pressure

We focused earlier (Chapter Seven) on some of our most devastating disorders. Included was a discussion of the almost-pandemic nature of cardiovascular disease and its relationship in reasonably well-controlled experiments to ascorbate supplementation. Limited studies were cited of the possible connection between one of, if not the most important, **prodromal** cardiovascular sign, namely hypertension. Hence, this is a good time to confirm the possible connection between vitamin C and blood pressure status.

In Chapter Nine mention was made of the celebrated NHANES I study. A data base of the National Center for Health Statistics, Health and Nutrition Examination Survey I (NHANES I) was used to perform a computer-assisted comprehensive analysis of the relation of 17 nutrients to the blood pressure profile of adult Americans. Subjects were 10,372 individuals, 18 to 74 years of age, who denied a history of hypertension and intentional modification of their diet. Incidentally, they employed the traditional criteria for high blood pressure, namely 140 over 90 mm Hg or greater as proposed by the American Heart Association.

According to McCarron and his associates at the Oregon Health Sciences University,[2] of the 17 dietary factors considered, they noted four were significantly related to the blood pressure state. Specifically, they observed that patients with high blood pressure were more prone to consume lesser amounts of calcium, potassium, vitamin A, and of particular relevance here, the ascorbates.

There are other individuals[3] who have examined the possible connection between vitamin C and blood pressure in somewhat more sophisticated systems. These researchers tested a group of healthy men (aged 30 to 39) to determine both their blood pressure (on the basis of the World Health Organizations criteria for hypertension) and their blood levels of ascorbic acid. They found that the higher the C levels, the lower the incidence of high blood pressure. These results, say the researchers, could help explain why some populations with high dietary intake of AA have a low mortality rate from heart disease and atherosclerosis, or hardening of the arteries.

These two reports make the point that there is reasonable evidence to show a significant correlation between ascorbic acid consumption and blood pressure. Within the limits of these studies, it's safe to conclude that those with hypertension appear to be the very same individuals with relatively poor vitamin C dietary intakes and marginally low blood vitamin C concentrations. While this information isn't proof positive, added to the earlier discussions (Chapter Seven), here is more data to encourage the need for ascorbic acid intake.

Arteriography: The Professed Gold Standard

Here we have an opportunity of comparing the agreed-upon-most sensitive measure of vitamin C metabolism versus the most critical diagnosis (except by experts in the field of nuclear medicine[4] of cardiovascular pathology.

One hundred fifty patients (100 males and 50 females) ages 19 to 78 with an average age of 51 years shared in this experiment.[5] They all had been referred for cardiologic consultation. Each had undergone cardiac catherization. The ascorbic acid level of the leukocytes in the patients with coronary artery disease (CAD) was compared to the vitamin C level of the leukocytes in the subjects without CAD as demonstrated by coronary arteriography.

We should mention that in traditional circles, the normal buffy coat concentration is approximately 25 to 50 mcg/10^8 (Chapter Four). Ramirez and Flowers from the University of Louisville, found that the leukocyte ascorbic acid level was markedly lower (17 mcg/10^8) in patients with coronary atherosclerosis as measured by this seeming gold standard.

Cancer Connections: An Overview

Among the most recent writings on the epidemiology of carcinomatosis and especially with regard to vitamin C, one must recognize the monumental work of Doctor Gladys Block. At the time of this publication, she was associated with the Division of Cancer Prevention and Control at the National Cancer Institute. This material was presented at a Conference on Vitamin C and Cancer which was held in

Washington, D. C. in 1990 and subsequently published in the *American Journal of Clinical Nutrition* in 1991.[6]

Epidemiologic evidence of a protective effect of ascorbic acid as judged in 11 non-hormone-dependent cancer sites is strong. Of the 46 such studies in which a dietary vitamin C index was calculated, 33 found statistically significant protection. High intake conferred a twofold insurance. Conversely, not one study was reported of a greater cancer risk with increased vitamin C intake.

In her own words:

> The strength and consistency of the results reported here for several sites suggests that there may be a real and important effect of ascorbic acid in cancer prevention.

Finally, Doctor Block very cautiously outlines the strengths and shortcomings of these epidemiologic trials. For example, she makes particular note of the paucity of studies of vitamin C in terms of serum and leukocyte concentrations.

One other document is described here because it attempts to recognize and obviate some of the objections raised by the report from the National Cancer Institute.

You will recall that on several occasions, the role of serendipity in vitamin C research reared its head. Here's another such case.

Researchers at the Albert Einstein College of Medicine in New York City were engaged in a study of vitamin A and its effect upon cervical dysplasia (a common precursor of cancer).[7] Quite by accident, they discovered some striking revelations about the ascorbates. They showed that women whose intake of vitamin C was less than 30 mg daily (only half the RDA and equal to about half a medium orange or two ounces of juice from concentrate) had a risk of developing cervical dysplasia ten times greater than that of women whose intake was higher. But we've gotten ahead of the story.

A case control study of women with cervical abnormalities identified through Pap smears, was conducted in the Bronx (New York) to explore the relationship between nutritional intake and cervical dysplasia. Nutrient consumption was estimated from computer analyses of three-day food records and 24-hour recall for 169 participants (87 cases, 82 controls), including a subset of 49 pairs matched for age, race and parity (number of children). Average vitamin C intake per day from three-day food records for controls was 107 mg compared to 80 mg for cases. Analysis of matched pairs showed similar results. Twenty-nine percent of cases compared to 3% of controls in matched subsets had vitamin C intake less than 50% of the RDA. This yielded a tenfold increase in risk of cervical dysplasia as estimated by odds ratio. The observations in this report are heightened by the fact that approximately one out of three US women in their reproductive years have daily vitamin C intake below 30 mg.

But let's not end without the caution delivered by these investigators:

> These data do not establish a cause-effect relationship between lower vitamin C intake and the development of cervical cancer. However, with the caveats noted, this dietary survey directs attention to a possible antioxidant role of vitamin C in the prevention of dysplastic progression identified with cervix cancer.

Finally, this information confirms the limited observations described earlier (Chapter Seven) regarding the possible role of vitamin C in carcinomatosis.

Insights into Vision

There's a bottom line to everything. The ultimate failure for the podiatrist is the amputation of the leg. The end of the line in dentistry is edentulousness. The checkmate for the vision scientist is blindness.

Interestingly, there are four major syndromes associated with sightlessness. The first has been mentioned earlier (Chapter Eight) in connection with diabetes mellitus. Consequently, it will not be discussed here. The other three are glaucoma, cataracts, and macular degeneration. (The latter will not be considered because of the sparse and fuzzy available information.) Hence, we will here consider only glaucoma and cataracts. Are there common connections and what role does vitamin C play?

Normalizing Eye Pressure

Professor Erik Linner at the University of Umea tells us of his and other studies dating back to the 1960s.[8] One experiment consisted of 25 glaucomatous people in their 60s who were provided 1/2 gram of vitamin C four times per day for six days. Following this oral treatment, the intraocular pressure decreased significantly 1.10 mm Hg.

The other experiment consisted of the topical application of a 10% aqueous solution of vitamin C to one eye utilizing the other eye as the control. This was carried out in 19 subjects with an average age of 63 for three days. Following this topical administration, the pressure in the test eye was significantly lower than that in the control eye.

Hence, within the limits of these two simple but well-designed experiments, one must conclude that beneficial effects can be found with the ascorbates. There's an additional point. This was accomplished with vitamin C eyedrops.

Yet another study was conducted by Michele Virno from the Eye Clinic at the University of Rome. Incidentally, he presented this paper at the Roman Ophthalmological Society in 1967 which was subsequently published.[9] In the main, he and his colleagues unlike Professor Linner emphasized the administration of the ascorbates by vein as well as orally. They also administered much larger dosages of vitamin C. In their own words:

> In all patients treated with a single oral dose (0.5 g/kg body weight) of vitamin C, a reduction in intraocular pressure was obtained . . . With repeated daily oral administration of vitamin C (the total amount of the drug being 0.5 to 0.7 g/kg body weight a day), it was possible to obtain almost normal tension levels in some patients whose intraocular pressure could not be controlled with . . . (the usual drugs).

Correcting Cataracts with C

Do you know that:

• 50 million people around the world at any one moment have cataracts?

• In the USA, 1.4 million, mostly elderly, had

cataract surgery in 1990?

• Medicare paid for 1.2 million of those extractions at a staggering cost of nearly $3.2 billion.

As far as we can determine, there are currently no clearly-designed double-blind studies of the causes of cataract formation. Only three serious epidemiologic reports are readily available.

It is generally conceded that biochemical evidence suggests that oxidative stress caused by accumulation of free radicals is involved in the pathogenesis of senile cataracts. If so, appropriate amounts of the antioxidant vitamins C and/or E might be expected to prevent or retard the process.

Here's a recent epidemiologic study by James Robertson and his group from the University of Western Ontario.[10] They very carefully looked at 175 cataract patients and compared them to 175 individually matched, cataract-free subjects. The most significant point is that they examined their consumption of supplementary vitamins. Specifically, the aim was to determine if subjects who were free of cataracts consumed more vitamins C and E than did a comparable group of people affected with the condition.

One of the unique features of this survey is that all interviews were conducted in the subjects' homes. Although this is more time consuming and expensive, it had the advantage of the respondents being more relaxed and open. An additional plus was that the participants were able to show the interviewers the drugs and vitamin preparations that they were taking. This is important because some 90% of the interviewees were aged 60 or over, a group in which recall is less efficient and "polypharmacy" is common.

Two points are obvious. First, cataract patients were only 30% as likely to have taken supplementary vitamin C. Secondly, the cataract-free subjects consumed approximately 300 to 600 mg of the ascorbates per day. (Once again, we find the desirableness of 300 to 400 mgs of C per day as cited earlier.)

The bare bones of this extraordinary survey can be summarized:

> . . . These results provide fair to good evidence for a causal association . . . This study suggests that the consumption of supplementary vitamins C and E may reduce the risk of senile cataracts by about 50-70% . . . Although most cataracts respond well to surgical treatment, this approach to even 50% of the combined prevalent and incident cases over the next five years would cost the Canadian health care system a minimum of $1.8 billion, based on an average cost per case of $3000.

The other epidemiologic study was conducted by Jacques and Chylack from Boston.[11] Their experimental design differed markedly from Robertson. None-the-less, the findings are quite in keeping with the earlier observations and simply expressed in their own conclusion:

> Subjects who consume fewer than 3.5 servings of fruit or vegetables per day had an increased risk of . . . cataracts.

Finally, in the interest of completeness, we should make note of a prospective study on nutrient intake and cataract extraction in women.[12] The objective was to examine the association between dietary intake of vitamin C and other nutrients. This study originated in 1980 and continued for eight years. It included subjects from 11 states. The participants (50,828) were female registered nurses 45 to 67 years of age. Apropos here is the fact that cataract formation was approximately 45% fewer in the subjects who employed vitamin C supplementation for a decade or more.

Summary and Conclusions

What makes this chapter unique is that we have largely examined correlative rather than straightforward causative data. So that the reader can better appreciate the intricacies of epidemiologic investigation, we have cited cardiovascular trends in the light of fresh fruits and vegetables. To say the least, there seems to be an exciting link.

This technique has been applied to problems previously discussed (e.g. cardiovascular disease and carcinomatosis) as well as syndromes not earlier considered (i.e. glaucoma and cataracts). The evidence presented here confirms the importance of vitamin C in those earlier disorders. Further, the data suggest also the utility of the ascorbates in the newer problems.

Vitamin C . . . who needs it? The data are reasonable to suggest that just about anybody with a medical problem would be well-served by considering additional ascorbate support.

Is vitamin C a panacea? Hardly. And the evidence that it is not a cure-all will become apparent in the next chapter.

14

MAN DOES NOT
LIVE BY C ALONE

Two points should be very clear. First, in a sense (and we brought this up in Chapter Two), vitamin C may be viewed like oxygen. When one discontinues air, death follows. Likewise, humans cannot manufacture vitamin C. Hence, when discontinued, there is certain cessation of vital functions. The major distinction is that with oxygen deprivation, death is quick . . . in minutes. In the case of the ascorbates, demise is slower . . . a matter of months or years.

It should not be surprising, as we have already learned from the earlier chapters that without ascorbic acid, there are inevitable medical problems.

It's easy to forget the flip side. One could take all the ascorbates in the world and still guarantee the very same mortality/morbidity because obviously man doesn't live by C alone!

The emphasis on the ascorbates may be likened to

clapping with one hand. Now we'll look at other possibilities, clapping with the other hand and with both. This will be accomplished with carefully executed trials with the bioflavonoids, the bioflavonoids plus the ascorbates, other antioxidants, and a potpourri of the remaining 40 plus nutrients.

Clapping with the Other Hand

In nature, vitamin C is more often than not packaged with one or more of a group of chemicals collectively referred as the bioflavonoids. For example, these substances in a grapefruit are disposed in the partitions that we eat between and leave behind. The story gets confusing because there are so many different names for the family members. You'll hear about the water soluble bioflavonoids, rutin, hesper, hesperiden, quercetin and many others. In the clinical environment, they're usually referred to as vitamin P. Some say that this label comes from the fact that the vitamin was early discovered in paprika. Others insist that the P means that the element plays a significant role in capillary permeability. (And we've already heard about the importance of small blood vessel health, Chapter Two.)

Notwithstanding the fact that it was discovered over 50 years ago, there is still confusion regarding its proper place in diet/nutrition and metabolism. As a matter of fact, according to the Tenth Revised Edition of the Recommended Dietary Allowances (RDAs), there is scarcely a word to emphasize its known utility and the suggested daily intake.

. . . Natural foods contain many compounds that have no known nutritional effects. These include the

167

flavonoids, rutin, quercetin, and hesperidin - the so-called vitamin P factors . . . [1]

For all of these reasons, we will now clap with the other hand and look at the role of the bioflavonoids in health and sickness.

Scoring Points with Vitamin P

Thus far, the experiments have been consistently those conducted in traditional universities, hospitals and other fancy centers by classical investigators.

The stories about to be told are special, if for no other reason than that they took place on a football field and a baseball diamond.

Of the many injuries associated with contact sports, the majority are sprains, strains and contusions. There is evidence in the literature that the bioflavonoids can, in some way, protect against these traumata. To evaluate the extent of this association, a double-blind study was conducted during the 1962 football season at Louisiana State University.[2]

Forty-eight players, including the 35 members of the varsity squad, were arranged randomly into two groups on a matched player basis. Throughout the pre-season practice and during the regular schedule each player received three soft gelatin capsules daily, two before the noon meal and the third at suitup time.

What this all means is that each student in this group was given 900 mg of the bioflavonoids each day. To the other group, a placebo (lactose formulation) was provided.

All injuries were carefully described and recorded as to location, type and severity at the time of occurrence. The most significant point is that the average recovery time per contusion was 10.5% longer for the placebo group. In other words, those given the bioflavonoids seemed to heal faster.

Using a more complicated formula, the sprains occurring in the bioflavonoid treated group were only three-fourths as severe as the placebo group. (The average recovery time per sprain was 18.9% longer for the placebo group.) However, the overall benefit of citrus bioflavonoid treatment reduced the duration of these injuries by 23%.

To get it perfectly clear, in their own words:

> This double-blind controlled evaluation of citrus bioflavonoids demonstrates their effect in improving the recovery rate of contusion and sprain injuries. The outstanding feature of the data presented is the significant reduction in the occurrence (58%) and severity of sprain injuries in the group on citrus bioflavonoids.

The story of bioflavonoids in sports medicine doesn't end on the football field. Professional baseball players are forever plagued with injuries. Regardless of the player's position, muscle strains, bruises, skin abrasions and joint injuries occur frequently.

In this connection, the bioflavonoids have been studied by the Los Angeles Dodgers.[3] It is of particular note that the average recovery time from all injuries in the bioflavonoid treated groups was 54% less than the untreated control groups. Let Doctor Woods tell us what he found in 1965:

> Citrus bioflavonoids, daily intake of 525 mg reduced the overall injury time off by 65%, when compared to the untreated reference group of players.

Two points. We've just observed the beneficial effects of somewhere between 525 and 900 mg of the bioflavonoids with regard to contact sport injuries reported back in the 60s. One has to ask what would have happened had even larger amounts been used? Obviously the answer must await further study. And this leads to the second item. We mentioned earlier the general position of the RDAs.[1]

Clapping with Both Hands

If it is unwise to consider the ascorbates alone, it's just as injudicious to view independently the bioflavonoids. And so, why not clap with both hands? The answer is that, in nature, as we have pointed out earlier, they do seem to come packaged together. Hence, it will be interesting now to examine, in reasonably executed studies, the clinical effects of the ascorbates plus the bioflavonoids.

Those Devastating Canker Sores

We discussed (Chapter Nine) the relationship of stomatology and vitamin C. Unfortunately, we made it sound as if there is only one oral disease, periodontal pathosis. Not true, as we'll learn. Also, we now have the opportunity to examine the combined effects of the ascorbates and the bioflavonoids. We will do this by looking at a very common oral condition, highly resistant-to-treatment, variously tagged herpes, herpes simplex, fever blisters, canker sores, herpetic lesions.

G. T. Terezhalmy, et al, of the National Naval Dental Center studied the efficacy of a water-soluble bioflavonoid-ascorbic acid complex in the treatment of

50 episodes of recurrent herpes labialis (blisters/ulcers on the lips). Twenty occurrences were treated with a complex of 600 mg of bioflavonoids and 600 mg of ascorbic acid administered three times daily. (This means a total of 1800 mgs of each per day.) Twenty other experiences were treated with a complex of 1000 mg of bioflavonoids and 1000 mg of vitamin C administered five times daily. (In other words, a total of 5000 mgs of each per day.) In ten other instances, the treatment consisted of a lactose placebo.

The therapeutic regimen was maintained for three days after the recognition of the initial symptoms associated with recurrent herpes labialis. The complex was observed to reduce vesiculation (blistering) and to prevent the disruption of the vesicular membrane. The therapeutic measure was obviously initiated during the prodromal (before blister formation) stage of the disease process.

What does all this mean? Optimal remission of symptoms was observed in about four days with the 1800 mg dosage of the bioflavonoids/ascorbic acid complex. In other words, one can expect the best results from this dosage in two to six days. (There was no advantage in giving the 5000 mg regimen.)

Incidentally, this is the largest dosage of the ascorbates (and also the bioflavonoids) cited thus far in this monograph. By the way, it is comforting that no adverse reactions were reported by any of the patients who participated in this investigation.

Female Problems . . . The Young and the Old

One of the single and biggest problems in young

women is excessive menstrual flow (also referred to in medical circles as menorrhagia). C. A. B. Clemetson and his associate (who were at the time of their report in Saskatchewan) looked at this problem in a group of presumably otherwise healthy young women.[5] They were given 200 mg of ascorbic acid and 200 mg of bioflavonoids three times a day. In other words, each of the subjects in the experimental group received 600 mg of both of these preparations on a daily basis. The control patients were given an indistinguishable dummy preparation. The results were clear. Thirty-two out of 37 women displayed decreased blood loss when treated with the test capsules for two months, while only one out of 13 showed a similar improvement with the placebo capsules.

Two additional points should be underlined. In general, classical scurvy can be so-called cured in about a week. But these women, who were in no way scorbutic, often required two months of treatment. Also, their excessive bleeding tended to return within a month or so after active therapy was discontinued.

There are still problems later on . . .

For a significant segment of the female population, the menopausal years can be a nightmare. In many instances, the flushing and associated complaints can be controlled, at a price, by estrogen supplementation. The at-a-price is the carcinogen potential of the female sex hormone. So, it would be a great contribution if it were possible to create this estrogenic effect with none-strogenic techniques. The bioflavonoids have been identified as such a preparation. Here is the story of the use of ascorbic acid/bioflavonoid supplementation upon the clinical symptomatology associated with the menopause.

A total of 94 patients were studied, of whom 36 were surgically-induced (also called castrates) and 58 who had undergone physiologic (natural) menopause.[6] Their symptoms were catalogued as severe, moderate, and mild. The test substance consisted of 200 mg of bioflavonoids and 200 mg ascorbic acid in each tablet administered six times per day. And so, each subject received 1200 mg of both the bioflavonoids and ascorbic acid daily. For comparison studies, controlled drugs included calcium carbonate, the antipyretic salicylamide, and an estrogen. Each patient received one course of each drug for a month. The compounds were designated only by letter and were indistinguishable in appearance. The composition of the agents wasn't known to the investigators nor to the patients. The results were tabulated as relieved, moderated, or no effect.

Table 14.1

Effect of one month of therapy upon menopausal hot flashes in subjects with physiologic menopause		
	complete relief	partial improvement	total
vitamin C and bioflavonoids	67	21	88
estrogen	36	36	72
salicylamide	26	24	50
calcium carbonate	12	10	22

Table 14.1 summarizes the responses to the four therapeutic agents in terms of complete, partial and

total relief. An analysis showed the bioflavonoid/vitamin C (line 1) to be markedly superior to all the other test substances in the relief of this single complaint. Actually, 67% reported complete relief, 21% partial making an overall 88% success factor.

The Whole May be Greater than the Sum of its Parts

We have just observed some of the merits of the bioflavonoids without the ascorbates. We have also had an opportunity to note the benefits of the combination. Since these substances appear in nature together, is there any evidence that the whole may be greater than the sum of its parts?

P. J. Warter and his associates have been conducting a series of interesting studies in rheumatic arthritis patients.[7] In one case, they examined 20 subjects, dividing them into three groups. One subset received 100 mg hesperidin plus 50 mg ascorbic acid, twice daily. They utilized the capillary fragility test as a reflection of change. The greatest improvement occurred with combined bioflavonoid/ascorbate supplementation.

Two years later, Warter and his team[8] pursued this investigation in 40 rheumatoid patients. As they put it:

> In 90% of the rheumatoid arthritis cases we found that a combination of hersperidin, 50 mg, and ascorbic acid, 50 mg, was effective in restoring capillary fragility to a normal state.

It would seem that, from these studies, they confirmed the old cliche "That the whole is indeed greater than the sum of its parts!'

Brambel[9] has studied two thousand patients in the past eleven years and found that hesperidin and ascorbic acid decreased the incidence of hemorrhagic complications sometimes encountered during anticoagulant therapy. He found that hesperidin or ascorbic acid alone was less effective than the combination.

From what has just transpired, the evidence suggests that the bioflavonoids plus vitamin C produce more startling clinical benefits than one or the other alone. In addition, there have been other and confirming studies to indicate the greater bioavailability when clapping with both hands. A notable example is the work of Joe A. Vinson and Pratima Bose from the University of Scranton.[10] These researchers carried out several well-designed studies utilizing the ascorbates with and without a citrus extract containing some of the bioflavonoid fractions. In every instance, it was obvious that adding vitamin P made for higher and more enduring plasma levels of the ascorbates. In other words, the combination yielded a bigger bang!

Cancer and Antioxidants Revisited

Much attention has been relegated to vitamin C in cancer (Chapters Seven and Thirteen). Considerable notice has been accorded the antioxidant family. What remains to be examined is the fact that other antioxidants (minus C) can also exert significant effect upon disease in carefully controlled experimental studies. This report on the relationship of vitamin A to precancer is an excellent example.

John Johnson, in a postdoctoral project, and his group studied 40 patients collected from the University of Alabama School of Dentistry, University Tumor Clinic and the Birmingham Veterans Administration Hospital.[11] An attempt was made in this investigation to study, under double-blind conditions, the effects of vitamin A versus placebo on leukoplakia in terms of its quantitative, qualitative, and histologic course. It appears that there is reduction in size, favorable qualitative change in the lesion, and histologic evidence of improvement. No such changes were noted in the placebo group.

The Big Picture

Finally, here is a reasonably-well supervised analysis which broadens the notion that there's much more to diet/nutrition than the ascorbates.

J. C. Brocklehurst and his comrades at the Farnborough Hospital in Kent described their novel experimental design in 80 geriatric patients.[12]

> They were selected solely on the basis that they were expected to survive in the hospital for a year to complete the study and that they could open their mouths sufficiently to make full clinical examination possible.

Half of these aged patients received a mixed vitamin B complex (15 mg thiamine, 15 mg riboflavin, 50 mg nicotinamide, 10 mg pyridoxine) and ascorbate (200 mg) supplement daily. There is no question but that the treated group demonstrated clinical and biochemical evidence of marked improvement (even with these surprisingly small amounts of vitamins). What is equally significant is that the placebo supplemented subset actually deteriorated during this same period.

On the basis of this very simple and reasonably well-controlled experiment, it should be concluded that there is clear evidence of a vitamin deficiency in many elderly patients in long-stay hospitals. These individuals demonstrate classical clinical signs of deficiency states. The overall picture can be remarkably improved with the administration of very simple dosages of other vitamins in combination with the ascorbates.

Summary and Conclusions

In the final analysis, there are approximately 40 plus nutrients. Hence, it is impossible to examine these many trillions of combinations.

On a more realistic plane, we have looked at some of these combinations. Certainly, in nature there's a marriage of the bioflavonoids and the ascorbates. This union has many worthwhile clinical benefits. But, more importantly, they are synergistic so that the whole is indeed greater than the sum of its parts. However, there are other antioxidants which contribute handily to health/sickness. The prime point of the matter is that man does not live by C alone!

So, what is the bottom line question that everybody is asking? *How much vitamin C should I take?* We'll look into this in the next and final chapter.

15

HOW MUCH VITAMIN C SHOULD I TAKE?

What all of us would like to know is the magic number. There is none for the same reason there's no one universal shoe size. And that all stems from the obvious . . . people are different.

Then What is There?

We've already raised the issue of the nature/nurture debate (Chapter Eleven). So, the role of genetics is obvious. It may be the basis for, in one case, a large stomach; in another instance, a small thyroid. These inherited properties certainly play a role . . . they modify vitamin C needs.

And then, we are also a product of our nurture. Surely, on the basis of size, a 200 pound healthy male needs more ascorbate than a 100 pound healthy woman. Clearly, our usual diets make a difference.

Some of us are meateaters; others vegetarians. A recent study by the National Cancer Institute found that 40% of Americans don't eat a single fruit and one out of five omit vegetables on a typical day. And then there are many other factors, some of which haven't and won't be mentioned such as pregnancy/lactation, lack of stomach acid, radiation, psychologic stressors, physical activity and sleep deprivation. It shouldn't be surprising that our AA wants are a function of the air we breathe, the water we drink, the foods we eat, the thoughts we have, and all else that is part and parcel of our lifestyle.

How Things Really Are

A survey of the databases for over-the-counter (OTC) and prescription preparations makes it crystal-clear that drugs are big business.[1]

• On average, your doctor will prescribe a drug every other time you see him/her.

• Up to half of the 1.6 billion prescriptions dispensed annually in the United States are used incorrectly.[2]

We have already examined (Chapter Ten) the risk/benefits of psychotherapeutic medications. You will recall a simple scoring system of pluses (benefits) and minuses (hazards). In Table 15.1 are listed six commonly employed prescription and OTC drugs clearly identified as modifying vitamin C state. In general, there are a small number of indications (as judged by the pluses). For example, in the case of one of our most popular contraceptive pills (Ortho-Novum) there are forty-six times more reasons for avoiding than using this agent.

Table 15.1

Reasons for and against common and representative drugs (expressed by number of lines of text)

drugs	pluses	minuses	approximate minus/plus ratio
Ortho-Novum (for birth control)	10	460	46
Advil (for kids)	13	321	25
Ecotrin (enteric-coated aspirin	12	80	7
terracycline (for infections)	18	107	6
Exedrin	4	19	5
Alka-Seltzer	8	32	4

But, more appropriately, what are the known connections between the ascorbates and such toximolecular medicinals? Are some of the unfavorable consequences of drugs (expressed in minuses) in some way connected with the ingestion, digestion, absorption, utilization, and/or excretion of vitamin C? Does the use of any of these thousands of commonly employed drugs change the answer to the question, "How much vitamin C should I take?"

Antibiotics . . . At What Cost?

It has long been recognized that the ascorbic acid content of **polymorphonuclear** cells bears a direct relationship to their phagocytic activity. We earlier discussed this call-to-arms (Chapter Six). Apropos, Shah and his associates at the Sarabhai Chemicals Research Institute in Ahmedabad studied the effect of tetracycline administration on the AA content in the plasma and in the leucocytes (buffy coat).[3] Fifteen healthy volunteers were divided into two groups, A and B, with ten and five individuals respectively. Both subsets received a 250 mg capsule of tetracycline four times a day for four days. Group B, in addition, was also provided at these same times with a 250 mg vitamin C pill.

The results are clear. In the tetracycline-only group there was a gradual fall in ascorbic acid levels of plasma as well as that of buffy coat. However, when tetracycline with ascorbates was administered, there was not only not a decline but, in fact, a convincing increase in blood levels.

Precisely how far reaching are these findings? In Table 15.1 (line 4), we discovered there are six times more lines of minuses (107) versus pluses (18). What we don't have is the intermediary connection between the Shah experiment and the findings in Table 15.1.

However, there is the more-than-circumstantial-evidence that many drugs behave in this very same fashion.

And so, how much vitamin C should I take? If you are one of the many millions on antibiotics, you might give serious thought to an ascorbic acid fortification program.

Aspirin has its Headaches

The salicylates (known to most of us as aspirin) in its many forms is a trademark of Americana. By act, if not by word, they are generally viewed as not only helpful but fortunately harmless. Table 15.1 lists several members of the salicylate family. The minus/plus ratios make it clear that this group is not without its problems.

In this connection, it is noteworthy that the Food and Drug Administration in a statement in 1990 will now be requiring labeling on all oral and rectal over-the-counter aspirin-containing products with a warning similar to that presently required on cigarettes![4]

What happens when one provides healthy young women with aspirin versus aspirin/ascorbate supplementation? Fourteen women, 22-28 years old, were studied by T. K. Basu at the University of Surrey in England.[5] First, he confirmed that the concentrations of vitamin C in plasma, leucocytes and urine are markedly elevated at various intervals following administration of a single oral dose of 500 mg of the ascorbates (Chapter Four). What he also reported was that the addition of aspirin (900 mg) in some way interfered with the absorption and utilization of vitamin C. For example, when aspirin was added to the C, only half as much appeared in the urine.

And so, how much vitamin C should I take? For the millions who "live on aspirin" and contribute to the 16,000 tons consumed annually in the USA, it might be well to consider the addition of the ascorbates.

What a Price for a Pill!

The happy news, of course, is that "the pill" prevents pregnancy. Unhappily, this is made possible at a price . . . by creating an unnatural state of perpetual pseudopregnancy. But the price is all of its attendant complications. For the record, check Table 15.1. For one of the popular oral contraceptive agents, Ortho-Novum (line 1), the benefits are expressed in ten lines. The minuses take up 460 lines . . . the unfavorableness is approximately 50 times greater! For many women the minuses are enough to make the pill just plain not worth it.

What does all this mean in terms of vitamin C needs?

The overwhelming concensus is that there's a definite connection. From the Department of Human Nutrition and Food of New York State College of Human Ecology at Cornell University, Jerry Rivers[6] — working alone and with Marjorie M. Devine[7]— noted decreased ascorbic acid concentrations in oral-contraceptive users as compared with controls.

Reduced levels were also observed by Victor Wynn of the Alexander Simpson Laboratory for Metabolic Research at Saint Mary's Hospital Medical School in London.[8] Wynn says that women using "the pill":

> . . . Would have to take about 500 mg of vitamin C daily to normalize blood and tissue levels.

As to increasing reports of adverse side effects and the controversy about risk/benefit ratio, we quote two researchers whose report was published in the distinguished scientific journal Nature. Michael and Maxine

Briggs[9] maintain:

> It is possible that some of the reported side-effects of "the pill" may be a consequence of this vitamin lack.

So, how much vitamin C should I take? For women who insist on this form of contraception, it looks from the evidence, that C supplementation is a must.

Let's Now Look at the Nondrug Drugs

We are dealing here with many other legal substances which aren't ordinarily recognized as drugs. Included in this category are tobacco (because of nicotine and other end-products), alcohol, coffee/tea, and many other caffeine-laden carbonated drinks. What these substances have in common is that they all contain drugs. For practical purposes, they are protoplasmic poisons.

- The average cup of brewed coffee contains about 85 mg of caffeine . . . just 14 mg less than a No-Doz pill.

- A Coke or a Tab has 24 mg . . . Excedrin, Anacin, Dristan and Sinarest each have about 30 mg of caffeine.

What's the relationship between these social/recreational drugs and vitamin C needs?

The Case of a Jigger of Booze

Guess . . . how many people in America drink alcohol? According to our best estimates, three out of four (including teenagers) use booze. Incidentally, there are only two countries on this planet, the Commonwealth of Independent States (the old Soviet Union) and Poland, which report greater guzzling than in these United States.

How does this influence the American Way? According to the U.S. Department of Health and Human Services, alcohol plays a role in:

• 37 of every 100 suicides

• 50% of all highway accidents

• approximately seven out of ten murders

• half of all arrests

• more mental-hospital admissions than for any other single cause

And what about the wallet? The National Institute on Alcohol Abuse and Alcoholism estimates:

• $10 billion in lost work time per annum

• $2 billion for the health and welfare of alcoholics and their families per year

• $3 billion in property damage, medical expenses, insurance costs and the like, year ly

• So, this amounts to a drain on the annual economy of $60 for every man, woman and child in America.

But, let's start at the beginning. What happens to vitamin C state with just one jigger of booze?

Virginia Fazio and her associates at the School of Sciences, Deakin University in Victoria, Australia were curious about this very question.[10] They took five people and studied the acute effects of alcohol on plasma ascorbic acid. After the ingestion of two grams of vitamin C and breakfast, plasma ascorbate rose two and a half fold in a matter of six hours. When 35 grams (a jigger) of alcohol was ingested with the two grams of AA and the same breakfast, plasma ascorbic acid consumption only doubled. The big difference persisted for the next 24 hours. To some, this may not sound like a big difference but extrapolate this to the real boozer who drinks much more and more often.

Lester and his associates at Yale University took the harder look at the bigger picture.[11] They examined the vitamin C needs of obvious alcoholics versus nonalcoholics by means of a so-called saturation test. This consisted of providing an oral ascorbate challenge and measuring the subsequent urinary excretion. (Incidentally, they reported an AA deficiency in 85% of 85 alcoholic patients on admission to the hospital.) Their results indicated that a 250 mg daily oral dose of ascorbic acid was insufficient to correct the initial deficit of the alcoholics in a seven-day period. In Doctor Lester's own words:

> . . . At least 500 mg of vitamin C daily for a week is required in alcoholic patients before placing them upon a maintenance regime.

So, how much vitamin C should I take? The many who consume alcohol might well find it worthwhile to consider a larger-than-usual AA program.

Smoke Gets in Your Blood
...Revisited

We have already learned (Chapter Three) that one of the major changes in the current RDA includes the recognition of a special need for more vitamin C in smokers. In addition, we and others have been examining the eating habits of tobacco consumers. For example, we, in our own laboratory, compared the dietary intake and nicotine habits in approximately 700 members of the health professions in 1975.[12]

Two observations are worthy of emphasis. It was found that, although the diets of both smokers and nonsmokers contained about the same number of calories, there was a great difference in the proportions of nutrients. On an average basis, for the smoker groups, the intake of almost every vitamin, mineral and amino acid studied was less than for the nonsmoker group.

The second observation consisted of the study of tobacco consumption in terms of vitamin C state and its effect upon oral symptomatology. The fewest oral findings were discovered with the least tobacco use and the highest AA intake (approximately 300 mg daily). Conversely, the greatest number of mouth symptoms and signs were noted in the heaviest smokers with also the poorest C diet.

Others have confirmed this diet/tobacco pattern.

Keith and Mossholder from the Department of Nutrition and Foods at Auburn University evaluated the nutritional status of a group of 11 smoking and 26 nonsmoking adolescent females (ages 14 to 17) with respect to vitamin C.[13] Dietary intakes of ascorbic acid were determined from two separate 24-hour food recalls. They came out with three notable conclusions. First, smokers consumed significantly less vitamin C than nonsmokers. Specifically, the daily intake in the smoker was 27 mg; the nonsmoker 73 mg. Hence, there was an approximate three-fold difference.

Second, the plasma level in the smoker was 0.3; in the nonsmoker 1.5. Thus, the difference is five times.

Finally, correcting for intake, when plasma AA values were adjusted for C consumption, smokers still exhibited a significantly lower plasma ascorbic acid concentration (0.5 mg/dl versus 1.4 mg/dl).

From these conclusions, it's safe to report that, for whatever reason, smokers tend to consume less of the ascorbates. Additionally, there are apparent differences in the absorption, assimilation, utilization, and/or excretion of the vitamin.

Schectman (you heard about him in Chapter Three) and his associates at the Medical College of Wisconsin in Milwaukee examined the findings of 11,592 respondents from the celebrated NHANES II survey.[14] They contribute additional information regarding number of cigarettes. For example, those smoking 20 or more cigarettes consumed 79 mg. Participants smoking one to 19 average 97 mg. Finally, no smokers ingested 107 mg. Thus, there is a neat and clean graded correlation. The greater the cigarette intake, the lower the ascorbic acid consumption. Serum vitamin C concentration was also examined. The heavy smokers (20+) had a serum of 0.8 mg/dl. The relatively mild consumers had 1.0 and the nonsmokers 1.2 mg/dl. Once again, the connection is clear. The poorest blood levels are in the heaviest smokers, the highest concentration in those who don't smoke.

Vitamin C . . . how much should I take? If you're a smoker, then you should give serious thought to increasing your ascorbic acid dietary and supplementation.

But, do we really know who is a smoker? It's becoming abundantly clear that many people not usually considered smokers, are unknowingly and/or involuntarily using this recreational drug. This is so because they live with, work with, or in some other way are intimately associated with a smoker. Therefore, they unwittingly or otherwise have the habit. These people obviously also need the ascorbate protection.

How and When . . . Vitamin C

One of the two final and burning questions is how and when the ascorbates should be administered.

In the surreal world, the answer is simple. We ought to pick the fresh fruits and vegetables off the trees and out of the ground. Frequent reference has been cited showing the relationships and benefits of vitamin C rich foods. Unfortunately, we live in a world where, for one of many reasons, it is no longer possible to live the simple life.

And so, there's a place for compromise. As for ascorbic acid, the tradeoff means taking this important nutrient in some concentrated form. As with all agents (even morphine) the intravenous route gives the biggest and quickest bang. Isolated studies have been reported in earlier chapters that underscore the utility for clinical and research purposes of IV ascorbic acid.

The end-results are less dramatic by intramuscular and the subcutaneous routes. Most of the evidence described in these chapters results from the simple oral administration of vitamin C. Finally, isolated instances have been cited for the use of the ascorbates in eye solutions, intranasal insufflation, and even by inunction (rubbing it on the skin).

Enough about the "how." What about the "when?"

Surprisingly little has been published. The sorriest way is throwing down all of the pills at one time (generally with hostility) and usually first thing in the morning. It is this way which has led to the oft-heard statement that taking vitamins is the best way of making expensive urine. What actually is more correct is that taking vitamins that way invites greater urinary excretion. From the limited work that has been done, it is suggested that the ascorbates be divided into several smaller amounts to be ingested periodically during the day. Since meals serve as markers, three or four times per day seems the reasonable "when" prescription.

Can You Take Too Much of a Good Thing?

Is it clinically possible? Of course, anything is possible. You can drink too much water (sometimes called drowning!). By the way, a report in the Journal of Emergency Medicine indicates data from the National Capitol Poison Center:

> Fatalities resulting from all major categories of prescription and nonprescription drugs during 1983-1989 was 1069. Fatalities from poisoning by vitamin supplements during that same time frame was 0!

Is it probable that you'll take too much? As we have seen time and time again throughout these pages, gram dosages of ascorbic acid proved to be beneficial for prevention and treatment. And you will recall, without any complications! Notwithstanding the evidence thus far, there are still alleged reports of kidney stones, systemic conditioning, uricosuria (uric acid in the urine), vitamin B_{12} destruction, mutagenicity (birth defects), and iron overload.

For the record, we have summarized the literature and our own experiences in two articles.[15,16] This has also been released in a full chapter entitled "Can Vitamin C Hurt You?"[17] But the most recent and complete summarization is available in a supplement of the International Journal for Vitamin and Nutrition Research.[18] And is well stated in the following:

> Despite contradictory reports the concensus from an extensive literature search is that these adverse health effects are not induced in healthy persons by ingesting large doses of ascorbic acid.

Of all the alleged clinical contraindications to megavitamin C, the only one, more a common inconvenience, is diarrhea. Taking too much C (whatever the amount may be) may cause loose stools. As a matter of fact, one can utilize bowel tolerance as a measure of how much vitamin C one needs. There's another plus. Since America is the most constipated country in the world, the diarrhea may actually be a blessing! So, there's very few serious "clinical" complications associated with so-called mega C.

But, what about the "biochemical" picture? On balance, the greatest amount of attention has been directed to the potential of oxalate crystals and kidney stones.

Here's a representative experiment based on fifty volunteers among the students and faculty of pharmacy at Ankara and Gazi Universities who were given two grams of vitamin C per day at regular time intervals for two months.[19] Blood and urine samples were collected in the beginning, one month and two months after vitamin administration. It will come as no surprise that blood and urine ascorbic acid levels were increased. But most importantly, the oxalates were not elevated.

And if this is not enough, Karl-Heinz Schmidt and his group from Germany, studied five healthy male volunteers.[20] Two grams of ascorbic acid were administered five times per day making a total daily intake of ten grams. Notwithstanding this large amount ingested, the increase in urinary oxalate was very low.

On the basis of these observations, along with the earlier cited reviews, one can conclude that ascorbic acid, even in relatively large amounts, is surprisingly safe.

So, How Much C Should I Take? Reprise

Just imagine, that the 250 million Americans are all of the same shape and size, living in an identical and incredible pristine and peaceful world. There would be a magic number. According to the National Research Council, it ought to be 60 mg of C per day. Cathcart, in his unusual report considers this the first face of vitamin C.[21] On the basis of our own observations as well as those derived from paleolithic man, the daily recommendation should be about 400 mg. This number seems to be reasonable for that theoretically healthy person living in that theoretically perfect world.

But look around. We're obviously not clones. Some are bigger and others smaller, fatter, thinner, smokers, contraceptive pill takers, aspirin and other drug consumers and on and on. These and other lifestyle characteristics color the answer to "How much C should I take?" From the experiments cited in this monograph as well as other literature, it looks like most of us would fare better if we consumed the ascorbates in daily gram amounts. Matthias Rath, M.D. (who has been mentioned earlier on several occasions) has looked at the optimal vitamin C intake through a study of cardiovascular health in guinea pigs with extrapolations to the human being. He presented his work at the Thirteenth International Conference on Human Functioning in 1992. In his opinion, the human equivalent for the ideal ascorbic acid intake is approximately 5,000 mg per day. This, as we have noted, is in keeping with the observations made and reported in a number of studies in this monograph. It is also consistent with the conclusions by Doctor Robert Cathcart in his discussions of the second face of the ascorbates.[21]

So, how big should the dosage be? There are three practical solutions.

For those who accept the "bowel tolerance theory," the answer is to increase ascorbic acid or its salts to the point just below diarrhea. For most Americans this would mean several grams when well and something more than that during stressful situations (e.g. during colds, serious illnesses). In the most fulminating of problems (i.e. AIDS, severe mononucleosis) the daily amounts acceptable by the human organism can be literally in hundreds of grams. In the Cathcart assignment, this is the third face of C.[21]

The second option is to answer the usual question, "What is vitamin C good for?" The World Health Organization has published a table of approximately 50 symptoms and signs in about 20 different sites. They're all non-specific. For example, metallic hair texture and easy bruisability are listed. The trick is to increase ascorbic acid until the relevant symptom and/or sign disappears.

For the more sophisticated, there are several tests (Chapter Four). Utilizing the most popular biochemical procedure, it would seem that a plasma vitamin C level of 1.0 mg% would be most desired. The optimal ranges have also already been cited for other procedures (Chapter Four). To attain these levels, most of us require several grams of the ascorbates per day.

Addendum ... At Long Last – (Some) Respect

In 1991, there appeared an interesting article in the prestigious professional journal *Science*[22] outlining the trials and tribulations of vitamin C from the 70s and Linus Pauling through the 1990s and Gladys Block. The author, Marcia Barinaga, with accuracy and appreciated charm and humor summarized the state of affairs:

> Researchers who work on vitamin C have something in common with comedian Rodney Dangerfield: They don't get much respect. At least they haven't until lately ... As more researchers begin looking into the chemical's potential ... Some say that the field is shedding its embarrasing past and achieving the respectability it has long been groping for ...

(Vitamin C) may play a role in chronic diseases such as cancer, heart disease, even AIDS . . . Like many scientific ideas once thought to be absurd that later appear in the guise of orthodoxy, vitamin C seems to be creeping closer and closer to winning the respect that Rodney Dangerfield never quite seems to get.

Obviously, the final word is not in. The professional pundits and the superscientific shamans will be arguing for a long time. While they do, what can we conclude? The approximately 100 studies including 50 well-designed, carefully-controlled, double-blind trials tell us that Mr. and Mrs. America could fare better than they do now with just a few grams of vitamin C daily. What do we mean by better? The evidence suggests that one can add significant years to life and obvious life to years! In the light of the favorable benefits/risks, what can we lose?

GLOSSARY

AA ≈ ascorbic acid

agglutination ≈ to clump

antimutagenic ≈ the factors which oppose change

ascorbate ≈ a salt of ascorbic acid (e.g. sodium ascorbate, calcium ascorbate)

ascorbic acid ≈ a substance, present in fresh green foods, citrus fruits, and various other uncooked materials, the lack of which in the body eventuallyleads to scurvy; also called vitamin C

biochemical ≈ the branch of chemistry that deals with plants and animals and their life processes

buffy coat layer ≈ a layer of white cells in the blood

capillary ≈ a microscopic blood vessel

carcinomatosis ≈ the existence of multiple cancers

collagen fibrils ≈ the fibers of a special kind of tissue found in bone and cartilage

collagen synthesis ≈ for formation of a specific type of tissue

cytogenetic ≈ cell formation

dorsum ≈ back

double blind ≈ denoting a manner of conducting an experiment so as to assure statistically reliable results, with neither experimenter nor subjects knowing what is used

ecchymosis ≈ passage of blood from ruptured blood vessels under the skin, marked by a purple dis-coloration

ecology ≈ the branch of biology that deals with the relations between living organisms and their environment

endogenous ≈ produced from within

erythrocytes ≈ the red blood cells

etiologic ≈ cause

fragility ≈ the capacity for being broken or destroyed

granulocytes ≈ one type of white blood cell

haemoglobin ≈ the red coloring matter of the red blood corpuscles; it carries oxygen from the lungs to the tissues and carbon dioxide from the tissues to the lungs, also spelled hemoglobin

hematocrit ≈ a popular and simple estimate of iron in the blood

hydroxylation ≈ a chemical phenomemon involving oxygen (0) and hydrogen (H). This important process is made possible in part by vitamin C.

hypercholesterolemia ≈ high blood cholesterol level

hypoascorbemic ≈ having low vitamin C levels in the blood

hypovitaminosis ≈ vitamin C deficiency

immunoglobulins ≈ proteins necessary in the immune system

integumentary ≈ skin

interferon ≈ one of many immune substances

intermediary ≈ go-between

intradermal ≈ between the layers of the skin

leukocytes ≈ the white blood cells

lingual ≈ tongue

mellitus ≈ a synonym for sweet or honey as in diabetes mellitus or sugar diabetes

metabolism ≈ the sum of the processes concerned in the building up and breaking down of living tissue

methylation ≈ a specific chemical process involving a group containing one carbon atom (C) and three hydrogen atoms (H)

monozygotic ≈ developed from a single fertilized egg or zygote, as in identical twins

mucosal pathosis ≈ disease of mucus membranes

myocardial infarction ≈ heart attack

neoplasma ≈ an abnormal new growth of tissue in animals or plants; frequently referred to as a tumor

nephrophy ≈ disease of the kidney

nonscorbutic syndromes ≈ the diseases and conditions generally not considered to be associ-ated with vitamin C deficiency

oxidation ≈ the chemical process by which oxygen (O) is combined with other chemical substances

pathology ≈ the branch of medicine concerned with the study of the nature of disease and conse-quences

peroxidation ≈ a process in which oxygen (O) is over added

petechia ≈ a small spot on a body surface, as the skin or mucous membrane, caused by a minute hemor-rhage

phagocytes ≈ a cell which engulfs or digests foreign bodies

pharmacology ≈ the branch of science that has to do with drugs in all their relations

physiologic ≈ the branch of biology dealing with the functions and vital processes of living organisms or their parts and organs.

platelet ≈ a minute piece of protoplasm circulating in the blood also called thrombocyte because of its importance in bleeding and clotting

polymorphonuclear ≈ most common type of white blood cell or phagocyte

prodromal ≈ early

prophylactic ≈ preventative

prostaglandins ≈ complex system of hormonelike substances

purpura ≈ a condition marked by purplish discolorations of the skin and mucous membranes caused by hemorrhages

red blood cell count ≈ the number of red blood cells (erythrocytes) per cubic millimeter of blood

rhinovirus (RV) ≈ one of a group of viruses of worldwide distribution which cause common colds

scorbutic ≈ another term for scurvy

seroconversion ≈ change in serum

serum AA ≈ blood ascorbic acid

sperm motility ≈ capacity of sperm to move

sperm volume ≈ quantity of sperm

stomatology ≈ medical study of the mouth

sulcus depth ≈ shallow crevice that normally surrounds a tooth

theobarbituric acid reactive substances ≈ too much or mismanaged oxygen

thromboatherosclerotic ≈ clotting in an artery that is hardening

thrombocytes ≈ blood platelets

volar ≈ front, or same side as the palm of the hand

REFERENCES

Chapter One

1. Coulter, H. L.
    The Controlled Clinical Trial.
    Washington, D. C., Center for Empirical Medicine. 1991.

2. Miller, J. Z., Nancy, W. E., Norton, J. A., Griffith,
    R. S., Rose, R. J., and Wolen, R. L.
    Therapeutic Effect of Vitamin C: A Co-Twin Control Study.
    Journal of the American Medical Association 237: #3, 248-251, 17 January
    1977.

3. Lewin, S.
    Vitamin C: Its Molecular Biology and Medical Potential.
    New York, Academic Press. 1976.

4. Cheraskin, E. and Ringsdorf, W. M., Jr.
    Biology of the Orthodontic Patient: I. Plasma Ascorbic Acid Levels.
    Angle Orthodontist 39: #2, 137-138, April 1969.

5. Cheraskin, E. and Ringsdorf, W. M., Jr.
    **Biology of the Orthodontic Patient: II. Lingual
    Vitamin C Test Scores.**
    Angle Orthodontist 39: #4, 324-325, October 1969.

6. Cheraskin, E. and Ringsdorf, W. M., Jr.
    Biology of the Orthodontic Patient: III. Relationship of Chronologic

and Dental Age in Terms of Vitamin C State.
Angle Orthodontist 42: #1, 56-59, January 1972.

7. Cheraskin, E. and Ringsdorf, W. M., Jr.
    Vitamin C and Chronologic Versus Bone Age.
    Journal of Oral Medicine 28: #3, 77-80, July-September 1973.

8. Burger, E. M., Tadiff, R. G., Scialli, A. R. and Zenick, H.
    Sperm Measures and Reproductive Success.
    New York, Alan R. Liss, Inc. 1989.

9. Behrman, S. J., Kistner, R. W. and Patton, G. W.
    Progress in Infertility, 3rd edition
    Boston, Little, Brown and Company. 1988.

10. Harris, W. A., Harden, T. E. and Dawson, E. B.
    Apparent Effect of Ascorbic Acid Medication on Semen Metal Levels.
    Fertility and Sterility 32: #4, 455-459, 1979.

11. Fraga, C. G., Motchnik, P. A., Shigenaga, M. K.,
    Helbock, H. J., Jacob, R. A. and Ames, B. N.
    Ascorbic Acid Protects Against Endogenous Oxidative DNA Damage in Human Sperm.
    Proceedings of the National Academy of Sciences 83: 11003-11006, December 1991.

12. Horowitz, J. M., Lafferty, E. and Thompson, D.
    The New Scoop on Vitamins.
    Time Magazine 139: #14, 48-53, 6 April 1992.

13. Suboticanec-Buzina, K., Buzina, R., Brubacher,
    G., Sapunar, J. and Christeller, S.
    Vitamin C Status and Physical Working Capacity in Adolescents.
    International Journal for Vitamin and Nutrition Research 54: #1, 55-60, 1984.

14. Clemetson, C. A. B.
    Vitamin C, 3 volumes.
    Boca Raton, CRC Press. 1989.

15. Ajayi, O. A. and Nnaji, U. R.
    Effect of Ascorbic Acid Supplementation on Haematological Response and Ascorbic Acid Status of Young Female Adults.
    Annals of Nutrition and Metabolism 34: #1, 32-36, 1990.

16. Cheraskin, E., Dunbar, J. B. and Flynn, F. H.
    The Intradermal Ascorbic Acid Test: Part I. A Review of Animal Studies.
    Journal of Dental Medicine 12: #4, 174-184, October 1957.

17. Dunbar, J. B., Cheraskin, E., and Flynn, F. H.
    The Intradermal Ascorbic Acid Test: Part II. A Review of Human Studies.
    Journal of Dental Medicine 13: #1, 19-40, January 1958.

18. Cheraskin, E., Dunbar, J. B., and Flynn, F. H.
    The Intradermal Ascorbic Acid Test: III. A Study of Forty-Two Dental Students.
    Journal of Dental Medicine 13: #3, 135-155, July 1958.

19. Dunbar, J. B., Cheraskin, E., Flynn, F. H. and Marley, J. F.
    The Intradermal Ascorbic Acid Test: IV. A Study of Tolerance Testing in Sixteen Dental Students.
    Journal of Dental Medicine 14: #3, 131-155, July 1959.

20. Ringsdorf, W. M., Jr. and Cheraskin, E.
    Intradermal Ascorbic Acid Test: Part V. Physiologic Range.
    Journal of Dental Medicine 17: #2, 76-79, April 1962.

21. Cheraskin, E., Ringsdorf, W. M., Jr., and Sisley, E. L.
    The Vitamin C Connection.
    New York, Harper & Row Publishers, Inc. (hardback) 1983.
    New York, Bantam Books, Inc. (paperback) 1984.

22. Cheraskin, E.
    The Vitamin C Controversy: Questions and Answers.
    1988. Wichita, Bio-Communications Press.

23. Delaney, L. and Ebbert, S.
    Reader-Tested Home Remedies: Second in a Five Part Series.
    Prevention Magazine 33-35, 104-110, January 1992.

Chapter Two

1. Rath, M.
   Solution to the Puzzle of Human Evolution.
   Journal of Orthomolecular Medicine 7: #2, 73-80,
   Second Quarter 1992.

2. Carpenter, K.J.
   The History of Scurvy and Vitamin C.
   1986. Cambridge, Cambridge University Press.

3. Jukes, T.H.
   The Identification of Vitamin C, an Historical Summary.
   Journal of Nutrition 118: #11, 1290-1293, November 1988.

4. Stone, I.
   The Healing Factor: Vitamin C Against Disease.
   New York, Grosset and Dunlap. 1972.

5. Pauling, L.
   Vitamin C and the Common Cold.
   San Francisco, W.H. Freeman and Company. 1970.

6. Pauling, L.
   Vitamin C, the Common Cold and the Flu.
   San Francisco, W.H. Freeman and Company. 1970.

7. Cameron, E.
   Hyaluronidase and Cancer.
   New York, Pergamon Press. 1966.

8. Cameron, E. and Pauling, L.
   Cancer and Vitamin C.
   Menlo Park, Linus Pauling Institute of Science and Medicine. 1979.

9. Eddy, T.P.
   A Study of the Relationship Between Hess Tests and Leucocyte Ascorbic Acid in a Clinical Trial.
   British Journal of Nutrition 27: #3, 537-542, May 1972.

10. Schultz, M.P.
    Studies of Ascorbic Acid and Rheumatic Fever II. Test of Prophylactic and Therapeutic Action of Ascorbic Acid.
    Journal of Clinical Investigation 15: 385-391, 1936.

Chapter Three

1. Levine, J.A. and Morgan, M.Y.
   Assessment of Dietary Intake in Man: A Review of Available Methods.
   Journal of Nutritional Medicine 2: #1, 65-81, 1991.

2. Food and Nutrition Board/Commission of Life Sciences/National Research Council.
   Recommended Dietary Allowances. Tenth, Edition. Washington, D.C., National Academy Press. 1989.

3. Patterson, B.H., Block, G., Rosenberger, W.F., Pee, D. and Kahle, L.L.
   Fruit and Vegetables in the American Diet: Data from the NHANES II

Survey.
American Journal of Public Health 80: #12, 1443-1449, December 1990.

4. Pelletier, O.
   Vitamin C Status of Cigarette Smokers and Nonsmokers.
   American Journal of Clinical Nutrition 23: #5, 520-524, May 1970.

5. Pelletier, O.
   Smoking and Vitamin C Level in Humans.
   American Journal of Clinical Nutrition 21: #10,
   1259-1267, October 1968.

6. Schectman, G., Byrd, J.C. and Hoffman, R.
   Ascorbic Acid Requirements for Smokers: Analysis of a Population Survey.
   American Journal of Clinical Nutrition 53: #6, 1466-1470, June 1991.

7. Ginter, E.
   Ascorbic Acid in Cholesterol Metabolism and in Detoxification of Xenobiotic Substances: Problem of Optimum Vitamin C Intake.
   Nutrition 5: #6, 369-374, November/December 1989.

8. Cheraskin, E., Ringsdorf, W.M., Jr., and Medford, F.H.
   The "Ideal" Daily Vitamin C Intake.
   Journal of the Medical Association of the State of Alabama 46: #12, 37-40,
   June 1977.

9. Cheraskin, E.
   The "Ideal" Vitamin C Intake.
   Journal of Orthomolecular Medicine 4: #1, 241, Fourth Quarter 1986.

10. Eaton, S.B., and Konner, M.
    Paleolithic Nutrition: A Consideration of its Nature and Current Implications.
    New England Journal of Medicine 312: #5, 283-288,
    31 January 1985.

Chapter Four

1. Buzina, R., Aurer-Kozelj, J., Srdak-Jorgic, D., Buhler, E., and Gey, K. F.
   Increase of Gingival Hydroxyproline and Proline by Improvement of Ascorbic Acid Status in Man.
   International Journal for Vitamin and Nutrition Research 56: #4, 367-372,
   1986.

2. Garry, P. J., Goodwin, J. S., Hunt, W. C., and Gilbert, B. A.
   Nutritional Status in a Healthy Elderly Population: Vitamin C.
   American Journal of Clinical Nutrition 36: #2, 332-339, August 1982.

3. Sauberlich, H. D.
    Implications of Nutritional Status on Human Biochemistry, Physiology, and Health.
    Clinical Biochemistry 17: 132-142, April 1984.

4. Schorah, C. J.
    Vitamin C Status in Population Groups.
    IN: Counsell, J. N. and Hornig, D. H.
    Vitamin C (Ascorbic Acid).
    Englewood, Applied Science Publishers. 1981.

5. Cheraskin, E., Dunbar, J. B. and Flynn, F. H.
    The Intradermal Ascorbic Acid Test: Part I. A Review of Animal Studies.
    Journal of Dental Medicine 12: #4, 174-184, October 1957.

6. Dunbar, J. B., Cheraskin, E., and Flynn, F. H.
    The Intradermal Ascorbic Acid Test: Part II. A Review of Human Studies.
    Journal of Dental Medicine 13: #1, 19-40, January 1958.

7. Dunbar, J. B., Cheraskin, E., and Flynn, F. H.
    The Intradermal Ascorbic Acid Test: Part IV. A Study of Tolerance Testing in Sixteen Dental Students.
    Journal of Dental Medicine 14: #3, 131-155, July 1959.

8. Cheraskin, E. and Ringsdorf, W. M., Jr.
    A Lingual Vitamin C Test: III. Relationship to Plasma Ascorbic Acid Level.
    International Journal for Vitamin Research 38: #1, 120-122, 1968.

9. Cheraskin, E. and Ringsdorf, W. M., Jr.
    A Lingual Vitamin C Test: XIX. Normal Versus Physiologic Range.
    Journal of the Ontario Dental Association 47: #10, 239-242, October 1970.

10. Cheraskin, E. and Ringsdorf, W. M., Jr.
    A Lingual Vitamin C Test: VI. Effect of Three Week Vitamin C Versus Placebo Supplementation.
    International Journal for Vitamin Research 38: #2, 257-259, 1968.

11. Cheraskin, E. and Ringsdorf, W. M., Jr.
    A Lingual Vitamin C Test: IV. Relationship to Intradermal Time.
    International Journal for Vitamin Research 38: #1, 123-126, 1968.

12. Sarji, K. E., Kleinfelder, J., Brewington, P., Gonzalez, J., Hempling, H. and Colwell, J. A.
    Decreased Platelet Vitamin C in Diabetes Mellitus: Possible Role in

Hyperaggregation.
Thrombosis Research 15: #5/6, 639-650, 1979.

13. Leggott, P. J., Robertson, P. B., Rothman, D. L., Murray, P. A. and Jacob, R. A.
Response of Lingual Ascorbic Acid Test and Salivary Ascorbate Levels to Changes in Ascorbic Acid Intake.
Journal of Dental Research 65: #2, 131-134, February 1986.

14. Clemetson, C. A. B.
Histamine and Ascorbic Acid in Human Blood.
Journal of Nutrition 110: #4, 662-668, April 1980.

Chapter Five

1. Johnston, C.S.
Effect of a Single Oral Dose of Ascorbic Acid on Body Temperature and Trace Mineral Fluxes in Healthy Men and Women.
Journal of the American College of Nutrition 9: #2, 150-154, April 1990.

2. Bordia, A. and Verma, S. K.
Effect of Vitamin C on Platelet Adhesiveness and Platelet Aggregation in Coronary Artery Disease Patients.
Clinical Cardiology 8: #10, 552-554, October 1985.

3. Aruma, O. I., Kaur, H., and Halliwell, B.
Oxygen Free Radicals and Human Diseases.
Journal of the Royal Society of Health 111: #5, 172-177, October 1991.

4. Moore, G. W., Strain, J. J., Nevin, G. B., Livingstone, B. E., Hannigan, B. M. and McKenna, P. G.
Blood and Urinary Measures of Oxidant Damage in Healthy Human Subjects.
Biochemical Society Transactions 18: 1168-1169, 1990.

5. Frei, B., England, L. and Ames, B. N.
Ascorbate is an Outstanding Antioxidant in Human Blood Plasma.
Proceedings of the National Academy of Sciences 86: 6377-6381, August 1989.

6. Fraga, C. G., Motchnik, P. A., Shigenaga, M. K., Helbock, H. J., Jacob, R. A. and Ames, B. N.
Ascorbic Acid Protects Against Endogenous Oxidative DNA Damage in Human Sperm.
Proceedings of the National Academy of Sciences 88: 11003-11006, December

1991.

7. Sram, R. J., Dobias, L., Pastorkova, A., Rossner, P. and Janca, L.
    Effect of Ascorbic Acid Prophylaxis on the Frequency of Chromosome Aberrations in the Peripheral Lymphocytes of Coal-Tar Workers.
    Mutation Research 120: #2&3, 181-186, May 1983.

8. Taylor, T. V., Rimmer, S., Day, B., Butcher, J., Dymock, I. W.
    Ascorbic Acid Supplementation in the Treatment of Pressure-Sores.
    Lancet 2: #7880, 544-546, 7 September 1974.

9. **Vitamin C Stabilizes Ferritin: New Insights into Iron-Ascorbate Interactions.**
    Nutrition Reviews 45: #7, 217-218, July 1987.

Chapter Six

1. Lewin, S.
    Vitamin C: Its Molecular Biology and Medical Potential.
    1976. New York, Academic Press.

2. Briggs, M.
    Vitamin C and Infectious Disease: A Review of the Literature and the Results of a Randomized, Double-Blind, Prospective Study Over 8 Years.
    IN: Briggs, M. H.
    Recent Vitamin Research.
    Boca Raton, CRC Press, Inc. 1984.

3. Prinz, W., Bortz, R., Bregin, B., and Hersch, M.
    The Effect of Ascorbic Acid Supplementation on Some Parameters of the Human Immunological Defense System.
    International Journal for Vitamin and Nutrition Research 47: #3, 248-257, 1977.

4. Anderson, R., Oosthuizen, R., Maritz, R., Theron, A. and Van Rensbrug, A. J.
    The Effects of Increasing Weekly Doses of Ascorbate on Certain Cellular and Humoral Immune Functions in Normal Volunteers.
    American Journal of Clinical Nutrition 33: #1, 71-76, January 1980.

5. Gotzsche, A.
    Pernasal Vitamin C and the Common Cold (Letter to the Editor).
    Lancet 2: #8670, 1039, 28 October 1989.

6. Carr, A. B., Einstein, R., Lai, L. Y. C., Martin, N. G. and Starmer, G. A.

Vitamin C and the Common Cold: Using Identical Twins as Controls.
The Medical Journal of Australia 2: #8, 411-412, October 1981.

7. Schultz, P. A., Dick, E. C., Mink, K. A., Norkus, E.,
    Olander, D., Jennings, L. C. and Inhorn, S. L.
    **Diminished Rhinovirus (RV) Illness Severity Correlates with
    Increased Leukocyte Ascorbic Acid (AA).**
    Journal of Infectious Diseases.
    Submitted for publication.

8. Cheraskin, E., Ringsdorf, W. M., Jr., Michael, D. W. and Hicks, B. S.
    Daily Vitamin C Consumption and Reported Respiratory Findings.
    International Journal of Vitamin and Nutrition Research 43: #1, 42-55, 1973.

9. Jewett, J. F. and Hecht, F. M.
    Preventive Health Care for Adults with HIV Infection.
    Journal of the American Medical Association 269: #9, 1144-1153, 3 March
    1993.

10. Cathcart, R. F., III
    A Unique Function for Ascorbate.
    Submitted for publication.

11. Cathcart, R. F., III
    **Vitamin C in the Treatment of Acquired Immune Deficiency
    Syndrome (AIDS).**
    Medical Hypothesis 14: #4, 423-433, August 1984.

12. Cathcart, R. F., III
    **Vitamin C: The Nontoxic, Nonrate-Limited, Antioxidant Free Radical
    Scavenger.**
    Medical Hypothesis 18: 61-77, 1985.

13. Harakeh, S., Jariwalla, R. J. and Pauling, L.
    **Suppression of Human Immunodeficiency Virus Replication by
    Ascorbate in Chronically and Acutely Infected Cells.**
    Proceedings of the National Academy of Sciences 87: #18, 7245-7249,
    September 1990.

14. Harakeh, S. and Jariwalla, R. J.
    **Comparative Study of the Anti-HIV Activities of Ascorbate and Thiol-
    Containing Reducing Agents in Chronically HIV-Infected Cells.**
    American Journal of Clinical Nutrition 54: 1231S-1235S, 1991.

15. McCormick, W. J.
    Ascorbic Acid as a Chemotherapeutic Agent.
    Archives of Pediatrics 69: #4, 151-155, April 1952.

Chapter Seven

1. Gunby, P.
    Battles Against Many Malignancies Lie Ahead as Federal "War on Cancer" Enters Third Decade.
    Journal of the American Medical Association 267: #14, 1891, 8 April 1992.

2. Rath, M. and Pauling, L.
    A Unified Theory of Human Cardiovascular Disease Leading the Way to the Abolition of This Disease as a Cause for Human Mortality.
    Journal of Orthomolecular Medicine 7: #1, 5-14, First Quarter 1992.

3. Rath, M.
    Solution to the Puzzle of Human Evolution.
    Journal of Orthomolecular Medicine 7: #2, 73-80, Second Quarter 1992.

4. Rath, M.
    Reducing the Risk for Cardiovascular Disease with Nutritional Supplements.
    Journal of Orthomolecular Medicine 7: #3, 153-162, Third Quarter 1992.

5. Van der Beek, E. J., van Dokkum, W., Schrijver, J., Wesstra, A. N., Kirtemaker, C., and Hermus, R. J. J.
    Controlled Vitamin C Restriction and Physical Performance in Volunteers.
    Journal of the American College of Nutrition 9: #4, 332-339, August 1990.

6. Osilesi, O., Trout, D. L., Ogunwole, J. O. and Glover, E. E.
    Blood Pressure and Plasma Lipids During Ascorbic Acid Supplementation in Borderline Hypertensive and Normotensive Adults.
    Nutrition Research 11: 405-412, 1991.

7. Bordia, A. K.
    The Effect of Vitamin C on Blood Lipids, Fibrinolytic Activity and Platelet Adhesiveness in Patients with Coronary Artery Disease.
    Artherosclerosis 35: #2, 181-187, February 1980.

8. Gore, J. M. and Dalen, J. E.
    Cardiovascular Disease.
    Journal of the American Medical Association 265: #23, 3105-3107, June 1991.

9. Block, G.
    Vitamin C and Cancer Prevention: The Epidemiologic Evidence.
    American Journal of Clinical Nutrition 53: 270S-282S, January 1991.

10. Cameron, E. and Pauling, L.
    Supplemental Ascorbate in the Supportive Treatment of Cancer: Prolongation of Survival Times in Terminal Human Cancer.
    Proceedings of the National Academy of Sciences 73: 3685-3689, 1976.

11. Cameron, E. and Pauling, L.
    Supplemental Ascorbate in the Supportive Treatment of Cancer: Reevaluation of Prolongation of Survival Times in Terminal Human Cancer.
    Proceedings of the National Academy of Science 75: 4538-4542, 1978.

12. Cameron, E. and Pauling, L.
    Cancer and Vitamin C.
    Menlo Park, Linus Pauling Institute of Science and Medicine. 1979.

13. Coon, W. W.
    Ascorbic Acid Metabolism in Postoperative Patients.
    Surgery, Gynecology, Obstetrics 114: #5, 522-534, May 1962.

14. U. S. Pharmaceutical Industry
    Annual Survey Report 1989-1991
    Pharmaceutical Manufacturers Association 26, October 1991.

15. Giles, W. H., Anda, R. F., Jones, D. H., Serdula, M. K., Merritt, R. K. and DeStefano, F.
    Recent Trends in the Identification and Treatment of High Blood Cholesterol by Physicians: Progress and Missed Opportunities.
    Journal of the American Medical Association 269: #9, 1133-1138, 3 March 1993.

Chapter Eight

1. Chesrow, E. J. and Bleyer, J. M.
   Results of Diabetes Detection Drives: With Special Reference to the Aged Population.
   Geriatrics 11: #3, 119-126, March 1956.

2. Danowski, T. S.
   Personal communication

3. Schappert, S. M.
   Office Visits for Diabetes Mellitus: United States, 1989.
   Advance Data from Vital and Health Statistics of the National Center for Health Statistics 211: 1-12, 24 March 1992.

4. Sigal, A. and King, C. G.
    The Relationship of Vitamin C to Glucose Tolerance in the Guinea Pig.
    Journal of Biochemical Chemistry 116: #2, 489-492, December 1936.

5. Cox, B. D. and Butterfield, W. J. H.
    Vitamin C Supplements and Diabetic Cutaneous Capillary Fragility.
    British Medical Journal 3: #5977, 205-207, 25 July 1975.

6. Ginter, E., Zdichynec, B., Holzerova, O., Ticha, T., Kobza, R., Sasko, E., and Gaher, M.
    Hypocholesterolemic Effect of Ascorbic Acid in Maturity-Onset Diabetes Mellitus.
    International Journal for Vitamin and Nutrition Research 48: #4, 368-373, 1978.

7. Cheraskin, E., Ringsdorf, W. M., Jr., Setyaadmadja, A. T. S. H. and Thielens, K. B.
    The Birmingham, Alabama, 1964 Diabetes Detection Drive: II. Age and Detrostix Patterns.
    The Alabama Journal of Medical Sciences 3: #2, 202-206, April 1966.

8. Setyaadmadja, A. T. S. H., Cheraskin, E., and Ringsdorf, W. M., Jr.
    Ascorbic Acid and Carbohydrate Metabolism: I. The Cortisone Glucose Tolerance Test.
    Journal of the American Geriatrics Society 13: #10, 924-934, 1965.

9. Davidson, M. B.
    Diabetes Mellitus: Diagnosis and Treatment, Third edition New York, Churchill Livingston. 1991.

10. Gambert, S. R.
    Diabetes Mellitus in the Elderly: A Practical Guide.
    New York, Raven Press. 1990.

11. Olson, O. C.
    Diagnosis and Management of Diabetes Mellitus, Second edition. New York, Raven Press. 1988.

12. Sperling, M. A.
    Physicians' Guide to Insulin-Dependent (Type 1) Diabetes Mellitus
    Alexandria, American Diabetes Association. 1988.

13. Bergman, M.
    Principles of Diabetic Management.
    New York, Medical Examination Publishing Company. 1987.

14. Dice, J. F. and Daniel, C. W.
    The Hypoglycemic Effect of Ascorbic Acid in a Juvenile-Onset
    Diabetic.
    Journal of the International Research Communications 1: #1, 41, March 1973.

15. Sylvest, O.
    The Effect of Ascorbic Acid on the Carbohydrate Metabolism.
    Acta Medica Scandinavia 110: #2-3, 183-196, 1942.

Chapter Nine

1. Russell, A. L.
   International Nutrition Surveys: A Summary of Preliminary Dental
   Findings.
   Journal of Dental Research 42: #1, 233-244, 1963.

2. Center for Disease Control
   Ten State Nutrition Survey, 1968-1970.
   Department of Health, Education, and Welfare Publication NO (HSM) 72-
   8131, Washington, D.C. Government Printing Office, 1972, pp. 87-93.

3. Ismail, A. I., Burt, B. A., and Eklund, S. A.
   Relation Between Ascorbic Acid Intake and Periodontal Disease in
   the United States.
   Journal of the American Dental Association 107: #6, 927-931, December 1983.

4. Council on Dental Therapeutics, American Dental Association.
   Accepted Dental Therapeutics, Edition 39
   Chicago, American Dental Association, pp. 137-138, 339. 1982.

5. Clark, J. W., Cheraskin, E., and Ringsdorf, W. M., Jr.
   An Ecologic Study of Oral Hygiene.
   Journal of Periodontology/Periodontics 40: #8, 476-480, August 1969.

6. El-Ashiry, G. M., Ringsdorf, W. M., Jr., and Cheraskin, E.
   Local and Systemic Influences in Periodontal Disease: II. Effect of
   Prophylaxis and Natural Versus Synthetic Vitamin C upon Gingivitis.
   Journal of Periodontology 35: #3, 250-259, May/June 1964.

7. El-Ashiry, G. M., Ringsdorf, W. M., Jr., and Cheraskin, E.
   Local and Systemic Influences in Periodontal Disease: III. Effect of
   Prophylaxis and Natural Versus Synthetic Vitamin C upon Sulcus
   Depth.
   New York Journal of Dentistry 34: #7, 254-262, August/September 1964.

8. El-Ashiry, G. M., Ringsdorf, W. M., Jr., and Cheraskin, E.
   Local and Systemic Influences in Periodontal Disease: IV. Effect of Prophylaxis and Natural Versus Synthetic Vitamin C upon Clinical Tooth Mobility.
   International Journal of Vitamin Research 34: #2, 202-218, 1964.

9. Leggott, P. J., Robertson, P. B., Rothman, D. L., Murray, P. A. and Jacob, R. A.
   The Effect of Controlled Ascorbic Acid Depletion and Supplementation on Periodontal Health.
   Journal of Periodontology 57: #8, 480-485, August 1986.

10. Cheraskin, E. and Ringsdorf, W. M., Jr.
    A Lingual Vitamin C Test: XV. A Predictor of Gingival Response to Oral Prophylaxis.
    International Journal for Vitamin Research 39: #1, 86-90, 1969.

11. Cheraskin, E., and Ringsdorf, W. M., Jr.
    A Lingual Vitamin C Test: XVI. A Predictor of Sulcus Depth Response to Oral Prophylaxis.
    International Journal for Vitamin Research 39: #1, 91-94, 1969.

12. Cheraskin, E.
    Vitamin C and Stomatology: A Mouthful of Evidence.
    Journal of Orthomolecular Medicine 6: #3&4, 147-154, Third and Fourth Quarter, 1991.

Chapter Ten

1. Cypress, B. K.
   Patients' Reasons for Visiting Physicians. National Ambulatory Medical Care Survey.
   Hyattsville, Maryland, United States Department of Health and Human Services, DHHS Publication No. (PHS) 82-1717. 1981.

2. Kinsman, R. A. and Hood, J.
   Some Behavioral Effects of Ascorbic Acid Deficiency.
   American Journal of Clinical Nutrition 24: #4, 455-464, April 1971.

3. McIntyre, J. S. and Romano, J.
   Is There a Stethoscope in the House (And is it Used)?
   Archives of General Psychiatry 34: #9, 1147-1151, September 1977.

4. Hall, R. C. W., Popkin, M. K., Devaul, R. A., Faillace, L. A. and Stickney, S. K.
   Physical Illness Presending as Psychiatric Disease.
   Archives of General Psychiatry 35: #11, 1315-1320, November 1978.

5. Hall, R. C. W.
    Psychiatric Presentations of Medical Illness: Somatopsychic Disorders.
    New York, SP Medical and Scientific Books. 1980.

6. Giurgea, C. E.
    Fundamentals to a Pharmacology of the Mind.
    Springfield, Charles C. Thomas. 1981.

7. Dean, W. and Morgenthaler, J.
    Smart Drugs and Nutrients.
    Santa Cruz, B & J Publications. 1990.

8. Goodwin, J. S., Goodwin, J. M. and Garry, P. J.
    Association Between Nutritional Status and Cognitive Functioning in a Healthy Elderly Population.
    Journal of the American Medical Association 249: #21, 2917-2921, 3 June 1983.

9. Schorah, C. J., Scott, D. L., Newill, A. and Morgan, D. B.
    Clinical Effects of Vitamin C in Elderly Inpatients with Low Blood-Vitamin C Levels.
    Lancet 1: #8113, 403-405, 24 February 1979.

10. Milner, G.
    Ascorbic Acid in Chronic Psychiatric Patients: A Controlled Trial.
    British Journal of Psychiatry 109: #459, 294-299, March 1963.

11. Naylor, G. J. and Smith, A. H. W.
    Vanadium: A Possible Aetiological Factor in Manic Depressive Illness.
    Psychological Medicine 11: 249-256, 1981.

12. *Physician's Desk Reference*
    Montvale, Medical Economics Data. 1992.

13. Barker, P. R., Manderscheid, R. W., Hendershot, G. E., Jack, S. S., Schoenborn, C. A. and Goldstorm, I.
    Serious Mental Illness and Disability in the Adult Household Population: United States, 1989.
    IN: *Advance Data*, Beltsville, Centers for Disease Control Number 218, 16 September 1992.

14. Jancar, J.
    Gradual Withdrawal of Tranquilizers with the Help of Ascorbic Acid.
    British Journal of Psychiatry 117: #537, 238-239, August 1970.

Chapter Eleven

1. Cheraskin, E.
   The Nature/Nurture Controversy: Spouse Likeness Revisited.
   Medical Hypotheses 33: #3, 219-225, November 1990.

2. Vinson, J. A., Chang, J. Y. and Nykaza, L.
   Effect of Ascorbic Acid Supplementation on Plasma Ascorbate and Lipid Peroxidation Parameters in Non-Smokers and Smokers.
   Medical Science Research 20: 483-484, 1992.

3. Young, R. W.
   Solar Radiation and Age-Related Macular Degeneration.
   Survey of Ophthalmology 32: #4, 252-269, January-February 1988.

4. Tappel, A. L.
   Will Antioxidant Nutrients Slow Aging Processes?
   Geriatrics 23: #10, 97-105, October 1963.

5. Tappel, A. L.
   Where Old Age Begins.
   Nutrition Today 2: #4, 2-7, December 1967.

6. Ames, B. N.
   The Causes and Prevention of Degenerative Diseases Associated with Aging.
   Personal communication.

7. Belloc, N. D. and Breslow, L.
   Relationship of Physical Health Status and Health Practices.
   Preventive Medicine 1: 409-421, 1980.

8. Wiley, J. A. and Camacho, T. C.
   Lifestyle and Future Health: Evidence from the Alameda County Study.
   Preventive Medicine 9: 1-21, 1980.

9. Enstrom, J. E., Kanim, L. D., and Klein, M. A.
   Vitamin C Intake Among a Sample of the United States Population.
   Epidemiology 3: #3, 194-202, May 1992.

10. Wilson, T. S., Weeks, M. M., Mukherjee, S. K., Murrell, J. S. and Andrews, C. T.
    A Study of Vitamin C Levels in the Aged and Subsequent Mortality.
    Gerontologia Clinica 14: #1, 17-24, 1972.

11. Schorah, C. J., Tormey, W. P., Brooks, G. H., Robertshae, A. M., Young, G. A., Talukder, R., and Kelly, J. F.

The Effect of Vitamin C Supplements on Body Weight, Serum
Proteins, and General Health of an Elderly Population.
American Journal of Clinical Nutrition 34: #5, 871-876, May 1981.

12. Bowers, E. F. and Kubik, M. M.
    Vitamin C Levels in Old People and the Response to Ascorbic Acid
    and to the Juice of Acerola.
    British Journal of Clinical Practice 19: #3, 141-147, March 1965.

13. Newton, H. M. V., Schorah, C. J., Nabibzadeh, N., Morgan,
    D. B. and Hullen, R. P.
    The Cause and Correction of Low Blood Vitamin C Concentrations in
    the Elderly.
    The American Journal of Clinical Nutrition 42: 656-659, October 1985.

Chapter Twelve

1. Dunbar, J. B., Cheraskin, E., Flynn, F. H. and Marley, J. F.
   The Intradermal Ascorbic Acid Test: Part IV. A Study of Tolerance
   Testing in Sixteen Dental Students.
   Journal of Dental Medicine 14: #3, 131-155, July 1959.

2. Ringsdorf, W. M., Jr. and Cheraskin, E.
   Vitamin C and Tolerance of Heat and Cold: Human Evidence.
   Journal of Orthomolecular Psychiatry 11: #2, 128-131, 1982.

3. Strydom, N. B., Korze, H. F., VanDerWalt, W. H. and Rogers, G. G.
   Effect of Ascorbic Acid on Rate of Heat Acclimatization.
   Journal of Applied Physiology 41: #2, 202-205, August 1976.

4. Nakamura, M., Kawagoe, T., Ogino, Y., Nishiyama, K.,
   Ichikawa, H. and Sugahara, K.
   Experimental Study on the Effect of Vitamin C on the Basal Metabolism
   and Resistance to Cold in Human Beings.
   Tohoky Journal of Experimental Medicine 92: #2, 207-219, June 1967.

5. Hindson, T. C.
   Ascorbic Acid for Prickly Heat.
   Lancet 1: #7556, 1347-1348, 22 June 1968.

6. Hindson, T. C. and Worsley, D. E.
   The Effects of Administration of Ascorbic Acid in Experimentally
   Induced Milaria and Hypohidrosis in Volunteers.
   British Journal of Dermatology 81: #3, 226-227, March 1969.

7. Ott, J. N.
   Health and Light.

1976. New York, Pocket Book.

8. Ott, J. N.
    Light, Radiation and You: How to Stay Healthy.
    1982. Old Greenwich, The Devin-Adair Company.

9. Darr, D., Combs, S., Dunston, S., Manning, T., and Pinnell, S.
    Topical Vitamin C Protects Porcine Skin from Ultraviolet Radiation-Induced Damage.
    British Journal of Dermatology 127: #3, 247-253, September 1992.

10. Murray, J., Darr, D., Reich, J., and Pinnell, S.
    Topical Vitamin C Treatment Reduces Ultraviolet B Radiation-Induced Erythema in Human Skin.
    Presentation before the Society of Investigative Dermatology.

11. Daniell, H. W.
    Smoker's Wrinkles: A Study in the Epidemiology of "Crow's Feet"
    Annals of Internal Medicine 75: #6, 873-880, December 1971.

12. Meisner, L.
    Personal communication.

13. Demis, D. J. and McGuire, J.
    Clinical Dermatology, Volume 2.
    Philadelphia, Harper and Row. 1984.

14. Lever, W. F. and Schaumburg-Lever, G.
    Histopathology of the Skin.
    Philadelphia, J. B. Lippincott Company. 1975.

15. Fitzpatrick, T. B., Eisen, A. Z., Wolff, K., Freedberg, I. M.,
    and Austen, K. F.
    Dermatology in General Medicine, 3rd edition.
    New York, McGraw Hill Book Company. 1987.

16. Wygarden, J. B. and Smith, M., Jr.
    Cecil Textbook of Medicine, 18th edition.
    Philadelphia, W. B. Saunders Company. 1988.

17. Sams, W. M., Jr., and Lynch, P. J.
    Principles and Practice of Dermatology.
    New York, Churchill Livingstone. 1990.

Chapter Thirteen

1. Verlangieri, A. J., Kapeghian, J. C., el-Deal, S., and Bush, M.

Fruit and Vegetable Consumption and Cardiovascular Mortality.
Medical Hypotheses 16: 7-15, 1985.

2. McCarron, D. A., Morris, C. D., Henry, H. J. and Stanton, J. L.
   Blood Pressure and Nutrient Intake in the United States.
   Science 224: #4656, 1392-1398, 29 June 1984.

3. Yoshioka, M., Matsushita, T. and Chuman, Y.
   **Inverse Association of Serum Ascorbic Acid Level and Blood Pressure
   or Rate of Hypertension in Male Adults Aged 30-39 Years.**
   International Journal for Vitamin and Nutrition Research 54: #4, 343-347,
   1984.

4. Ell, P. J.
   Nuclear Medicine.
   Postgraduate Medicine Journal 68: 82-105, 1992.

5. Ramirez, J. and Flowers, N. C.
   **Leukocyte Ascorbic Acid and Its Relationship to Coronary Artery
   Disease in Man.**
   American Journal of Clinical Nutrition 33: #10, 2079-2087, October 1980.

6. Block, G.
   Vitamin C and Cancer Prevention: The Epidemiologic Evidence.
   American Journal of Clinical Nutrition 53: #1, 270S-282S, January 1991.

7. Wassertheil-Smoller, S., Romney, S. L., Wylie-Rosett, J.,
   Slagle, S., Miller, G., Lucido, D., Duttagupta, C. and Palan, P. R.
   Dietary Vitamin C and Uterine Cervical Dysplasia.
   American Journal of Clinical Nutrition 144: #5, 714-724, November 1981.

8. Linner, E.
   **The Pressure Lowering Effect of Ascorbic Acid in Ocular
   Hypertension.**
   Acta Ophthalmologica 47: #2, 685-689, 1969.

9. Virno, M., Bucci, M. G., Pecori-Giraldi, J., and Missiroli, A.
   Oral Treatment of Glaucoma with Vitamin C.
   Eye, Ear, Nose and Throat Monthly 46: #12, 1502-1508, December 1967.

10. Robertson, J. M., Donner, A. P. and Trevithick, J. R.
    A Possible Role for Vitamins C and E in Cataract Prevention.
    American Journal of Clinical Nutrition 53: #1, 346S-351S, January 1991.

11. Jacques, P. F. and Chylack, L. T., Jr.
    **Epidemiologic Evidence of a Role for the Antioxidant Vitamins and
    Carotenoids in Cataract Prevention.**
    American Journal of Clinical Nutrition 53: #1, 352S-355S, January 1991.

12. Hankinson, S. E., Stampfer, M. J., Seddon, J. M., Colditz,
    G. A., Rosner, B., Speizer, F. E. and Willett, W. C.
    Nutrient Intake and Cataract Extraction in Women: A Prospective Study.
    British Medical Journal 305: #6849, 335-339, 8 August 1992.

Chapter Fourteen

1. Food and Nutrition Board/Commission of Life Sciences/
   National Research Council.
   Recommended Dietary Allowances, Tenth edition.
   Washington, D.C., National Academy Press, pp 262-263. 1989.

2. Broussard, M. J.
   Evaluation of Citrus Bioflavonoids in Contact Sports.
   Citrus in Medicine 2: #2, October 1963.

3. Woods, R. M.
   Effects of Citrus Bioflavonoids in Professional Baseball.
   Citrus in Medicine 3: #1, 102, February 1965.

4. Terezhalmy, G. T., Bottomley, W. K., and Pelleu, G. B.
   The Use of Water-Soluble Bioflavonoids-Asorbic Acid Complex in the Treatment of Recurrent Herpes Labialis.
   Oral Surgery, Oral Medicine, and Oral Pathology 45: #1, 56-62, January 1978.

5. Clemetson, C. A. B. and Blair, L. M.
   Capillary Strength of Women with Menorrhagia.
   American Journal of Obstetrics and Gynecology 83: #10, 1269-1279, May 1962.

6. Smith, C. J.
   Non-Hormonal Control of Vaso-Motor Flushing in Menopausal Patients.
   Chicago Medicine, 7 March 1964.

7. Warter, P. J., Drezner, H. L. and Horoschak, S.
   Effect of Hesperidin and Ascorbic Acid on Capillary Fragility in Rheumatic Arthritis.
   Journal of the Medical Society of New Jersey 43: 228-230, 1946.

8. Warter, P. J., Drezner, H. L. and Horoschak, S.
   Influence of Hesperidin-C on Abnormal Capillary Fragility in Rheumatic Arthritis Patients.
   Delaware State Medical Journal 20: #3, 41-45, March 1948.

9. Brambel, C. E.

The Role of Flavonoids in Coumarin Anticoagulant Therapy.
Annals of the New York Academy of Sciences 61: #3, 678-683, 8 July 1955.

10. Vinson, J. A. and Bose, P.
    Comparative Bioavailability to Humans of Ascorbic Acid Alone or in a Citrus Extract.
    American Journal of Clinical Nutrition 48: #3, 601-604, September 1988.

11. Johnson, J. E., Ringsdorf, W. M., Jr. and Cheraskin, E.
    Relationship of Vitamin A and Oral Leukoplakia.
    Archives of Dermatology 88: #5, 607-612, November 1963.

12. Brocklehurst, J. C., Griffiths, L. L., Taylor, G. R., Marks, J., Scott, D. L., and Blackley, J.
    The Clinical Features of Chronic Vitamin Deficiency: A Therapeutic Trial in Geriatric Hospital Patients.
    Gerontologia Clinica 10: #5, 309-320, 1968.

Chapter Fifteen

1. Cheraskin, E.
   Human Health and Homeostasis: VI. Drugs and Homeostatic Process.
   The International Journal of Biosocial and Medical Research 13: #2, 200-210, December 1991.

2. Bulletin
   Working to Improve the Safe and Effective Use of Prescription Medicines.
   National Council on Patient Information and Education, Washington, D.C.

3. Shah, K. V., Barbhaiya, H. C. and Srinivasan, V.
   Ascorbic Acid Levels in Blood During Tetracycline Administration.
   Journal of Indian Medical Association 51: #3, 127-129, August 1968.

4. Food and Drug Administration
   New Warning Label for Over-the-Counter Aspirin.
   Journal of the American Medical Association 264: #6, 677, 8 August 1990.

5. Basu, T. K.
   Vitamin C-Aspirin Interactions.
   IN: Hanck, A.
   Vitamin C: New Clinical Applications in Immunology, Lipid Metabolism, and Cancer.
   1982. Bern, Hans Huber Publishers.

6. Rivers, J. M.
   Oral Contraceptives and Ascorbic Acid.

American Journal of Clinical Nutrition 28: #5, 550-554, May 1975.

7. Rivers, J. M. and Devine, M. M.
    Plasma Ascorbic Acid Concentrations and Oral Contraceptives.
    American Journal of Clinical Nutrition 25: #7, 684-689, July 1972.

8. Wynn, V.
    Vitamins and Oral Contraceptive Use.
    Lancet 1: #7906, 561-564, 8 March 1975.

9. Briggs, M. and Briggs, M.
    Vitamin C Requirements and Oral Contraceptives.
    Nature 238: #5362, 277, 4 August 1972.

10. Fazio, V., Flint, D. M., and Wahlzvist, M. L.
    Acute Effects of Alcohol on Plasma Ascorbic Acid in Healthy Subjects.
    American Journal of Clinical Nutrition 34: #1, 2394-2396, November 1981.

11. Lester, D., Buccino, R. and Bizzocco, D.
    The Vitamin C Status of Alcoholics.
    Journal of Nutrition 70: #2, 278-282, February 1960.

12. Cheraskin, E., Ringsdorf, W. M., Jr., and Medford, F. H.
    Eating Habits of Smokers and Nonsmokers.
    Journal of the International Academy of Preventive Medicine 11: #2, 9-17,
    Second Quarter, 1975.

13. Keith, R. E. and Mossholder, S. B.
    **Ascorbic Acid Status of Smoking and Nonsmoking Adolescent
    Females.**
    International Journal for Vitamin and Nutrition Research 56: 363-366, 1936.

14. Schectman, G., Byrd, J. C. and Gruchow, H. W.
    The Influence of Smoking on Vitamin C Status in Adults.
    American Journal of Public Health 79: #2, 158-162, February 1989.

15. Ringsdorf, W. M., Jr. and Cheraskin, E.
    **Medical Complications from Ascorbic Acid: A Review and
    Interpretation (Part One).**
    Journal of Holistic Medicine 6: #1, 49-63, Spring/Summer, 1984.

16. Ringsdorf, W. M., Jr. and Cheraskin, E.
    **Medical Complications from Ascorbic Acid: A Review and
    Interpretation (Part Two).**
    Journal of Holistic Medicine 6: #2, 173-183, Fall/Winter 1984.

17. Cheraskin, E., Ringsdorf, W. M., Jr, and Sisley, E. L.
    The Vitamin C Connection.

1983. New York, Harper and Row Publishers, Inc. (hardback) pp 201-219.
1984. New York, Bantam Books, Inc. (paperback) pp 221-240.

18. Rivers, J. M.
    Safety of High-Level Vitamin C Ingestion.
    International Journal of Vitamin and Nutritional Research (supplement) 30:
    95-102, 1989.

19. Erden, F., Hacisalihoglu, A., Kocer, Z., Simsek, B.,
    Nebioglu, S.
    **Effects of Vitamin C Intake on Whole Blood Plasma, Leucocyte and
    Urine Ascorbic Acid and Urine Oxalic Acid Levels.**
    Acta Vitaminology and Enzymology 7: #1-2, 123-130, 1985.

20. Schmidt, K., Hagmaier, V., Hornig, D. H., Vuilleumier,
    J. P. and Rutishauser, G.
    **Urinary Oxalate Excretion After Large Intakes of Ascorbic Acid in
    Man.**
    American Journal of Clinical Nutrition 34: #3, 305-311, March 1981.

21. Cathcart, R. F., III.
    The Third Face of Vitamin C.
    The Journal of Orthomolecular Medicine 7: #4, 197-200, Fourth Quarter,
    1992.

22. Barinaga, M.
    Vitamin C Gets a Little Respect.
    Science 254: #5030, 374-376, 18 October 1991.

Dr. Emanuel Cheraskin, a leading authority on scientific measurement and data acquisition, has contributed to over five hundred publications in a distinguished fifty-year career. The precision of his results and the exacting nature of his procedural technique have sealed his reputation as one of the twentieth century's most respected empirical analysts.

Dr. Cheraskin was awarded his M.D. from the University of Cincinnati College of Medicine and his D.M.D. from the University of Alabama School of Dentistry. He and his wife presently enjoy at least one daily glass of orange juice on a balcony overlooking the hills of Alabama.